Veterinary Embryology

NIPA® GENX ELECTRONIC RESOURCES & SOLUTIONS P. LTD.
New Delhi-110 034

About the Editor

Dr. Tanmoy Rana obtained his Bachelor of Veterinary Sciences and Animal Husbandry degree (B.V.Sc. & A.H.) and Masters (M.V.Sc) in Veterinary Medicine, Ethics & Jurisprudence from West Bengal University of Animal and Fishery Sciences, Kolkata, India. He secured his Doctor of Philosophy (Ph.D.) in Veterinary Science from the University of Calcutta, Kolkata, India. He works currently as an Assistant Professor of the Veterinary Clinical Complex at West Bengal University of Animal and Fishery Sciences, Kolkata, India. Previously he has also worked as a Veterinary Officer, Animal Resources Development Department, Government of West Bengal, India. He is actively engaged in teaching and clinical practices in veterinary medicine and research related to animal health, production, and disease monitoring regimes. His research interests involve arsenic toxicity, molecular diagnosis, molecular toxicology and medicine, oxidative stress, immunopathology, nanoparticles, Echinococcosis, and microbes. He has published several research articles in reputed international and national journals along with review articles in international journals. He is an editorial board member (especially BMC Veterinary Research, Associate Editor of Frontier in Veterinary Science), and a reviewer of international and national journals. He is a member of many international scientific societies and organizations importantly the West Bengal Veterinary Council (WBVC), The Indian Society for Veterinary Medicine (ISVM), the Association of Public Health Veterinarians, and The Indian Science Congress Association (ISCA). He is also an associate of the West Bengal Academy of Science & Technology, West Bengal, India. He is an editor and author of so many national and international books.

Veterinary Embryology

Tanmoy Rana, Ph.D.
AFWAST, FVASc., Assistant Professor
Veterinary Clinical Complex
(Veterinary Medicine, Ethics & Jurisprudence)
Department of Veterinary Clinical Complex
West Bengal University of Animal & Fishery Sciences
Kolkata-700037, West Bengal, India

NIPA® GENX ELECTRONIC RESOURCES & SOLUTIONS P. LTD.
New Delhi-110 034

NIPA® GENX ELECTRONIC RESOURCES & SOLUTIONS P. LTD.

101,103, Vikas Surya Plaza, CU Block
L.S.C. Market, Pitam Pura, New Delhi-110 034
Ph : +91-11-43860225, Mob.: +91 9717133558, 9540816132
E-mail: newindiapublishingagency@gmail.com
Website: www.nipaersources.com

Print ISBN: 978-93-58873-25-2
ebook ISBN: 978-93-58871-68-5

NIPA® also publishes books in a variety of electronic formats. Some content that appears in print may not be available in electronic books, and vice versa.

Composed and Designed by NIPA®.

Preface

Notes on Veterinary Embryology 1e. Is structured for the better knowledge and understanding of Veterinary Embryology. The multiple choice question book (MCQ) provides MCQ of development of all organ systems, including important molecular aspects of animal development. Book chapters of the book are written by a large team of competent authors with extensive experience of teaching this subject in a user-friendly way. The book describes a short note of the development stages of all organs with MCQ for the students and job aspirants especial preparing for various examination like ICAR-JRF, SRF, NET, ARS, CSIR/ICMR-JRF, UPSC, State PSCs, PG and PhD Entrance and other competitive exams. The MCQ book is carefully written on the short notes of general aspect of development from formation of the gametes, through fertilization and initial embryogenesis with organ formation and thereby special developmental stages of the organ system with MCQ for the evaluation. MCQs on teratology and assisted reproduction technologies were also provided in the book. Students of animal science, veterinary medicine, biomedical sciences and biotechnology, at both undergraduate and postgraduate stages of their careers, will find this book essential for their needs. This book will be immensely useful and adds resources to all students of veterinary college, academicians, paper setters, job aspirants. I think the book remains an important resource for the competitive examination. I hope the book helps the reader immensely.

Tanmoy Rana
Department of Veterinary Clinical Complex
West Bengal University of Animal & Fishery Sciences
Kolkata, India

Acknowledgement

I convey my sincere gratitude to the Hon'ble Vice Chancellor, West Bengal University of Animal & Fishery Sciences for providing me with the opportunity to edit the book. I also thank all contributors who wrote the manuscript and sent it in time. I am really indebted to all colleagues for their useful ideas, constant help, and suggestions for the improvement of the book. I am really helpful to all members of the publisher for helping me a lot for editing the book. Lastly, I am also grateful to family members for providing a great support and the time to finalize the book.

Tanmoy Rana
Department of Veterinary Clinical Complex
West Bengal University of Animal & Fishery Sciences
Kolkata, India

Contents

1

General Introduction

Monalisha Debbarma[1], Mohamed Hasif Ganimattoullah[2] and Tanmoy Rana[3]

[1]Department of Veterinary Anatomy and Histology, Institute of Veterinary Science and Animal Husbandry, Siksha O Anusandhan University, Odisha

[2]Department of Veterinary Physiology, Institute of Veterinary Science and Animal Husbandry, Siksha O Anusandhan University, Odisha

[3]Department of Veterinary Clinical Complex, West Bengal University of Animal & Fishery Sciences, Kolkata

Introduction

Veterinary embryology is a fundamental branch of veterinary science that focuses on the study of the development of embryos in animals, tracing the journey from the moment of fertilization to the point where a fully developed fetus is formed. This field is not just an academic endeavor but a critical component of veterinary practice, research, and animal husbandry. It offers profound insights into the origins of life, the complex processes that drive the formation of tissues and organs, and the ways in which genetic and environmental factors interact to shape the development of an organism.

The field of veterinary embryology is vast and encompasses several stages of development. The process begins with gametogenesis, where the reproductive cells—sperm in males and ova in females—are produced through a process of meiosis. These gametes are haploid, meaning they contain half the number of chromosomes found in somatic cells. The union of these gametes during fertilization restores the diploid number of chromosomes, marking the beginning of a new individual organism. The fertilized egg, or zygote, is the starting point of embryonic development.

Following fertilization, the zygote undergoes a series of rapid cell divisions known as cleavage. During cleavage, the single-celled zygote divides without growing, resulting in a cluster of smaller cells called blastomeres. This process continues until the formation of a structure known as the blastocyst, which consists of an inner cell mass that will eventually develop into the embryo, and an outer layer of cells called the trophoblast, which will form the placenta. The blastocyst is a critical stage in development as it is involved in implantation into the uterine wall, a necessary step for establishing a successful pregnancy.

The next major phase in embryonic development is gastrulation, a highly orchestrated process that results in the formation of three primary germ layers: the ectoderm, mesoderm, and endoderm. These layers are the foundation for all the tissues and organs in the body. The ectoderm gives rise to the nervous system, skin, and sensory organs; the mesoderm forms the skeletal system, muscles, circulatory system, and kidneys; while the endoderm develops into the gastrointestinal tract, liver, pancreas, and lungs. Gastrulation is a critical step in embryogenesis, as it establishes the basic body plan of the organism.

Following gastrulation, organogenesis begins—the process by which the germ layers differentiate into specific organs and tissues. This stage is marked by the formation of the neural tube, which will become the central nervous system, and the development of the heart and circulatory system, which are among the first organs to function. The complexity of organogenesis highlights the intricate coordination of genetic and molecular signals that guide cells to adopt specific fates and form functional structures. Errors in this process can lead to congenital malformations, which underscores the importance of understanding the mechanisms of normal development.

Veterinary embryology is not limited to the study of normal development but also includes the investigation of developmental abnormalities and congenital defects. Understanding the causes of these anomalies, which can be genetic, environmental, or a combination of both, is crucial for developing preventive and therapeutic strategies in veterinary medicine. For instance, certain genetic mutations can result in hereditary conditions that are passed down through generations, while environmental factors, such as exposure to toxins or nutritional deficiencies, can interfere with normal embryonic development.

The knowledge gained from veterinary embryology has practical applications in various fields, including animal breeding, reproductive technologies, and conservation biology. In animal husbandry, for example, understanding the principles of embryology is essential for improving reproductive efficiency and managing breeding programs. Techniques such as artificial insemination, in vitro fertilization (IVF), and embryo transfer are all grounded in the principles of embryology. These techniques not only enhance the genetic quality and productivity of livestock but also help preserve endangered species by facilitating reproduction in controlled environments.

In addition to its applications in agriculture, veterinary embryology plays a crucial role in the field of regenerative medicine and genetic engineering. Advances in stem cell research, for example, are closely linked to embryological studies, as stem cells are derived from early embryonic cells. These pluripotent cells have the potential to differentiate into various cell types, making them invaluable for developing therapies to repair damaged tissues or treat degenerative diseases. Genetic engineering, on the other hand, involves manipulating the genome of an organism at the embryonic stage to introduce desirable traits or correct genetic defects. This technology holds great promise for improving animal health and productivity, as well as for producing transgenic animals that can serve as models for human diseases or as bioreactors for producing pharmaceuticals.

Conservation biology also benefits from the insights provided by veterinary embryology. Many species are at risk of extinction due to habitat loss, climate change, and human activities. Assisted reproductive technologies, such as IVF and cloning, offer new hope for preserving genetic diversity and preventing the extinction of endangered species. By studying the embryonic development of these species, scientists can develop strategies to improve their reproductive success in captivity and reintroduce them into the wild)

Veterinary embryology also intersects with the field of veterinary pathology, where the study of embryonic and fetal development aids in diagnosing and understanding the causes of reproductive failures, miscarriages, and stillbirths. In this context, embryology provides the framework for investigating the impact of diseases, infections, and toxic exposures on the developing embryo. For instance, certain infectious agents can cross the placental barrier and cause congenital infections, leading to developmental abnormalities or fetal death. By identifying these pathogens and understanding their effects on embryonic development, veterinarians can devise strategies to prevent and manage such conditions.

Furthermore, veterinary embryology contributes to the advancement of animal welfare. Understanding the needs and vulnerabilities of embryos at different stages of development can help improve the conditions under which animals are bred and raised. For example, optimizing the environment for pregnant animals can reduce the risk of prenatal stress, which has been shown to affect embryonic development and long-term health outcomes for the offspring. In addition, knowledge of embryology is crucial for refining techniques such as embryo transfer, ensuring that the procedure is as safe and effective as possible.

In summary, veterinary embryology is a multifaceted field that encompasses the study of the earliest stages of life in animals. It provides essential insights into the processes that govern development, from fertilization to the formation of a fully functional organism. The knowledge gained from this field has wide-ranging applications in veterinary medicine, animal husbandry, conservation, regenerative medicine, and animal welfare. By understanding the principles of embryology, veterinarians and researchers can improve reproductive success, prevent congenital diseases, and contribute to the health and well-being of animals across a variety of species. The continued study of veterinary embryology is vital for advancing our understanding of life's origins and for addressing the challenges faced by the animal populations that share our planet.

Multiple Choice Questions

1. Developmental anatomy is concerned with:
   a) Only pre-natal development
   b) Only post-natal development
   c) The formative history from fertilization to maturity
   d) The study of diseases in adults
2. The study of different developmental processes in various species is known as:
   a) Functional Embryology b) Comparative Embryology
   c) Morphological Embryology d) Experimental Embryology
3. Ontogeny refers to:
   a) Evolutionary history of a species
   b) Development from fertilization to maturity
   c) The study of different species' embryonic stages
   d) The comparison of developmental stages across species
4. The concept that "ontogeny repeats phylogeny" suggests:
   a) Embryos follow evolutionary history during development
   b) Evolutionary history is not reflected in embryonic development
   c) Phylogenetic traits are not observed in ontogeny
   d) All species have identical developmental stages

5. The process by which the zygote undergoes repeated cell division is known as:
   a) Cleavage
   b) Gastrulation
   c) Organogenesis
   d) Differentiation
6. What does the term "pluripotent" describe?
   a) Cells that can form any tissue type
   b) Cells with limited developmental potential
   c) Cells that are capable of forming any organ
   d) Cells capable of forming various specialized tissues
7. Amniotes are characterized by:
   a) Fertilization occurring outside the body
   b) Development within an amniotic cavity
   c) Lack of amniotic fluid
   d) Direct nutrient transfer from maternal blood
8. Anamniotes are:
   a) Animals with internal fertilization
   b) Animals that develop in an amniotic sac
   c) Animals with external fertilization
   d) Mammals with live births
9. Viviparous animals:
   a) Lay eggs that develop outside the body
   b) Develop embryos within an amniotic sac
   c) Have embryos that develop inside the body with nutrient transfer via placenta
   d) Do not undergo internal fertilization
10. The structure that provides nourishment to the embryo in birds and reptiles is called:
    a) Amniotic fluid
    b) Placenta
    c) Yolk
    d) Decidua
11. The term "deutoplasm" refers to:
    a) The outer layer of the blastula
    b) The inner layer of the gastrula
    c) The reserve food material in ova
    d) The early stage of the embryo
12. The term "totipotent" describes:
    a) Cells that can only form specific tissues
    b) Cells that can form an entire organism
    c) Cells that cannot form new individuals
    d) Cells that are differentiated
13. The process of forming three germ layers (ectoderm, mesoderm, endoderm) is known as:
    a) Cleavage
    b) Gastrulation
    c) Organogenesis
    d) Differentiation

14. The primary germ layers are:
    a) Ectoderm, Mesoderm, Endoderm
    b) Epidermis, Dermis, Hypodermis
    c) Epiblast, Hypoblast, Mesoblast
    d) Outer layer, Inner layer, Middle layer
15. Which theory explains that cells in the embryo become functionally and biochemically different during development?
    a) Germ plasm theory b) Mosaic theory
    c) Regulative theory d) Differentiation
16. The event where cells or tissues regenerate lost parts is called:
    a) Metamorphosis b) Growth
    c) Regeneration d) Differentiation
17. The duration from fertilization to birth is referred to as:
    a) Gestation period b) Incubation period
    c) Neonatal period d) Pre-pubertal period
18. The "decidua" is:
    a) The fertilized ovum
    b) The reserve food material in ova
    c) The modified endometrium after implantation
    d) The outer layer of the blastula
19. The phase of development where organs and systems are formed is:
    a) Cleavage b) Gastrulation
    c) Organogenesis d) Metamorphosis
20. The scientist known as the Father of Modern Embryology is:
    a) Aristotle b) Karl Ernst Von Baer
    c) William Harvey d) Hans Driesch
21. The term "neonatal" refers to:
    a) The period from birth to sexual maturity
    b) The period from fertilization to birth
    c) The period from birth to physiological adaptation
    d) The period after puberty
22. The scientist who first observed sperm cells was:
    a) Antonie van Leeuwenhoek b) Karl Ernst Von Baer
    c) William Harvey d) Franz von Leydig
23. Which of the following is NOT a phase of ontogenic development?
    a) Gametogenesis b) Cleavage
    c) Regeneration d) Adaptation

24. The process where embryos develop new structures in response to injury is known as:
    a) Metamorphosis
    b) Asexual reproduction
    c) Regeneration
    d) Growth
25. The "gestation period" refers to:
    a) The time period from birth to sexual maturity
    b) The duration from fertilization to birth
    c) The time period of development in an egg
    d) The period of physiological adaptation post-birth
26. The process by which the blastula transforms into the gastrula with three distinct layers is:
    a) Organogenesis
    b) Cleavage
    c) Gastrulation
    d) Differentiation
27. The term "epigenesis" describes:
    a) The embryo being preformed in the egg
    b) The formation of new organs during development
    c) Development as a gradual process with successive organ formation
    d) The inheritance of traits through gametes
28. The term "adult" refers to:
    a) The stage before puberty
    b) The stage following the cessation of reproduction
    c) The period of sexual maturity and reproductive capability
    d) The period from birth to physiological adaptation
29. The stage in development characterized by significant increases in cell number and size is:
    a) Cleavage
    b) Organogenesis
    c) Growth
    d) Metamorphosis
30. The event where an embryo starts developing specialized functions and structures is known as:
    a) Differentiation
    b) Gastrulation
    c) Cleavage
    d) Growth
31. The fully developed female sexual cell is termed:
    a) Ovum
    b) Spermatozoon
    c) Zygote
    d) Blastula
32. In vertebrates, the size of the egg chiefly depends on:
    a) Its shape
    b) The amount of yolk reserves
    c) The age of the female
    d) The environmental conditions
33. Typically, the mature eggs are:
    a) Spherical in shape
    b) Cuboidal in shape
    c) Elongated
    d) Disc-shaped

34. The primary egg membrane that develops around the plasma membrane of the egg is known as:
   a) Vitelline membrane
   b) Chorion
   c) Albumen
   d) Calcareous shell
35. Secondary egg membranes are produced by:
   a) The ovum itself
   b) The follicle cells surrounding the oocyte
   c) The oviducts
   d) The surrounding water
36. The tertiary egg membrane that includes the albumen is found in:
   a) Mammals
   b) Birds and reptiles
   c) Insects
   d) Amphibians
37. The egg membrane consisting chiefly of calcium carbonate is called:
   a) Vitelline membrane
   b) Calcareous shell
   c) Jelly envelope
   d) Zona pellucida
38. The type of egg with a small amount of yolk is termed:
   a) Microlecithal
   b) Mesolecithal
   c) Macrolecithal
   d) Discoidal
39. The egg type where yolk is concentrated in the center is called:
   a) Isolecithal
   b) Telolecithal
   c) Centrolecithal
   d) Discoidal
40. The main axis of an egg connects:
   a) The animal pole and the vegetal pole
   b) The egg membrane and the cytoplasm
   c) The nucleus and the yolk
   d) The egg white and the yolk
41. Fertilization is the union of which two gametes?
   a) Spermatozoon and ovum
   b) Spermatozoon and zygote
   c) Ovum and blastula
   d) Spermatozoon and egg cell
42. Internal fertilization is typical in:
   a) Amphibians
   b) Insects
   c) Mammals
   d) Echinoderms
43. The enzyme produced by sperm to penetrate the egg's corona radiata is:
   a) Hyaluronidase
   b) Lysin
   c) Fertilizin
   d) Acrosin
44. The acrosome reaction involves:
   a) Fusion of sperm and egg membranes
   b) Breakdown of the sperm tail
   c) Formation of the fertilization cone
   d) Release of lysins

45. The formation of the fertilization cone is associated with:
    a) Activation of the ovum
    b) Capacitation
    c) Sperm and egg fusion
    d) Barrier penetration
46. Monospermy describes fertilization by:
    a) Multiple sperm
    b) One sperm
    c) No sperm
    d) Any number of sperm
47. Pathological polyspermy results in:
    a) Normal development
    b) Abnormal development
    c) Enhanced genetic variation
    d) Increased fertility
48. In which type of egg is the yolk distributed unevenly, concentrated at one end?
    a) Isolecithal
    b) Telolecithal
    c) Centrolecithal
    d) Discoidal
49. The egg membrane that is formed by the ovum itself is classified as:
    a) Secondary
    b) Tertiary
    c) Primary
    d) None of the above
50. The term for the area of the egg with the most yolk concentration is:
    a) Animal pole
    b) Vegetal pole
    c) Equatorial region
    d) Blastodisc
51. The process by which sperm become capable of fertilization is called:
    a) Capacitation
    b) Activation
    c) Fusion
    d) Amphimixis
52. The type of polyspermy where only one sperm participates in embryo development is:
    a) Pathological
    b) Physiological
    c) Natural
    d) Artificial
53. The formation of the fertilization membrane occurs during:
    a) Sperm and egg fusion
    b) Activation of the ovum
    c) Barrier penetration
    d) Migration of pronuclei
54. The zona pellucida is an example of:
    a) A tertiary egg membrane
    b) A primary egg membrane
    c) A secondary egg membrane
    d) An accessory layer
55. In which type of egg is the yolk concentrated at the center, with a small layer of cytoplasm around it?
    a) Isolecithal
    b) Telolecithal
    c) Centrolecithal
    d) Discoidal
56. The term "vitelline membrane" refers to:
    a) A secondary egg membrane
    b) A tertiary egg membrane
    c) A primary egg membrane
    d) An external shell layer

57. The process where the sperm and egg nuclei combine to restore the diploid state is called:
    a) Capacitation b) Amphimixis
    c) Fertilization d) Activation
58. The acrosome reaction is essential for:
    a) Egg activation b) Fertilization cone formation
    c) Capacitation d) Sperm-egg fusion
59. Which structure helps keep the egg cell in the center of the egg white?
    a) Chalazae b) Zona pellucida
    c) Vitelline membrane d) Calcareous shell
60. In which type of egg is the yolk scattered evenly throughout the cytoplasm?
    a) Isolecithal b) Telolecithal
    c) Centrolecithal d) Discoidal
61. The structure that provides nutrition to the developing embryo is the:
    a) Animal pole b) Vegetal pole
    c) Yolk sac d) Acrosome
62. The term "discoidal eggs" refers to eggs with:
    a) Evenly distributed yolk
    b) Yolk concentrated in a disc-shaped area
    c) Small amounts of yolk
    d) Yolk distributed at the poles
63. Which type of fertilization occurs in most terrestrial animals?
    a) External b) Internal
    c) Artificial d) Natural
64. The zona radiata is found in:
    a) Secondary egg membranes b) Primary egg membranes
    c) Tertiary egg membranes d) None of the above
65. The term for the reaction that makes the egg membrane resistant to multiple sperm entry is:
    a) Acrosome reaction b) Cortical reaction
    c) Capacitation d) Fertilization reaction
66. The stage of development characterized by cleavage, morula formation, and blastocyst implantation is called:
    a) Germinal stage b) Embryonic stage
    c) Foetal stage d) Blastula stage
67. During which stage do the three germinal layers differentiate and most tissues and organs form?
    a) Germinal stage b) Embryonic stage
    c) Foetal stage d) Morula stage

68. The foetal stage is primarily characterized by:
   a) Tissue differentiation
   b) Growth of various systems and placenta development
   c) Cleavage and blastocyst formation
   d) Morula formation
69. The gestation period for a cow ranges from:
   a) 280 to 290 days b) 330 to 340 days
   c) 60 to 65 days d) 110 to 130 days
70. Which animal has the longest gestation period?
   a) Cow b) Elephant
   c) Rhinoceros d) Human
71. The spherical shape of the embryo during late cleavage stage is called:
   a) Blastula b) Morula
   c) Blastocyst d) Zygote
72. The stage after the morula, where the embryo forms a hollow sphere of cells, is known as:
   a) Blastula b) Cleavage
   c) Morula d) Gastrula
73. What is the cavity inside the blastula called?
   a) Yolk sac b) Blastocoel
   c) Amniotic cavity d) Chorionic cavity
74. The process where the embryo attaches and embeds in the uterine wall is called:
   a) Blastulation b) Cleavage
   c) Implantation d) Fertilization
75. In which stage does the zona pellucida disappear to allow implantation to begin?
   a) Germinal stage b) Embryonic stage
   c) Foetal stage d) Blastocyst stage
76. Which cleavage pattern is characterized by cells arranged radially around the polar axis?
   a) Spiral cleavage b) Radial cleavage
   c) Bilateral cleavage d) Biradial cleavage
77. What is the cleavage pattern where the upper tier of cells is displaced sidewise over the lower cells?
   a) Spiral cleavage b) Radial cleavage
   c) Bilateral cleavage d) Biradial cleavage
78. Which type of cleavage involves divisions that only occur in a small amount of active cytoplasm around the egg?
   a) Holoblastic cleavage b) Meroblastic cleavage
   c) Superficial cleavage d) Discoidal cleavage

79. The type of blastula formed in holoblastic embryos with a central blastocoel is:
a) Stereoblastula b) Coeloblastula
c) Periblastula d) Discoblastula

80. Which type of blastula is characterized by a solid mass of cells with a very small blastocoel?
a) Stereoblastula b) Coeloblastula
c) Periblastula d) Discoblastula

81. In which type of egg does discoidal cleavage occur?
a) Isolecithal b) Mesolecithal
c) Telolecithal d) Centrolecithal

82. In which animal does implantation occur by adhesion and apposition rather than invasion?
a) Pigs b) Cows
c) Humans d) Horses

83. The trophoblast layer of the blastocyst differentiates into which two layers?
a) Cytotrophoblast and syncytiotrophoblast
b) Epiblast and hypoblast
c) Endoderm and ectoderm
d) Mesoderm and ectoderm

84. The bilaminar germ disc forms between which two cavities in the early blastocyst?
a) Primary yolk sac and primary amniotic cavity
b) Blastocoel and chorionic cavity
c) Amniotic cavity and chorionic cavity
d) Yolk sac and blastocoel

85. The process where trophoblastic cells invade the endometrial stroma with proteolytic enzymes is known as:
a) Implantation b) Cleavage
c) Morulation d) Blastulation

86. The part of the trophoblast that covers the embryonic pole of the blastocyst is known as:
a) Mural trophoblast b) Polar trophoblast
c) Syncytiotrophoblast d) Cytotrophoblast

87. During which stage does the embryo begin to form the germ layers?
a) Morula stage b) Blastocyst stage
c) Gastrula stage d) Foetal stage

88. Which type of cleavage is typical of a highly telolecithal egg, such as in birds?
a) Holoblastic b) Meroblastic
c) Superficial d) Discoidal

89. The term “epiblast” refers to:
   a) The outer layer of the bilaminar germ disc
   b) The inner layer of the bilaminar germ disc
   c) The layer of cells surrounding the yolk sac
   d) The trophoblast layer of the blastocyst

90. What is the main function of the amniotic sac during embryonic development?
   a) Provide nutrients
   b) Protect the embryo from mechanical injury
   c) Facilitate implantation
   d) Provide initial oxygen supply

91. Which type of cleavage pattern is associated with the development of a blastocyst in mammals?
   a) Radial cleavage
   b) Spiral cleavage
   c) Discoidal cleavage
   d) Holoblastic cleavage

92. The primary function of the chorion during early development is to:
   a) Form the placenta
   b) Protect the embryo from environmental stress
   c) Support the yolk sac
   d) Facilitate implantation

93. What structure forms from the inner cell mass of the blastocyst?
   a) Trophoblast
   b) Epiblast
   c) Cytotrophoblast
   d) Syncytiotrophoblast

94. The yolk sac plays a crucial role in:
   a) Oxygen exchange
   b) Nutrient supply
   c) Hormone production
   d) Immunity

95. What is the main function of the primary yolk sac in early development?
   a) Exchange of gases
   b) Providing nutrients to the developing embryo
   c) Forming the placenta
   d) Protecting the embryo from mechanical stress

96. Which animal is an example of eccentric implantation?
   a) Bitch
   b) Mouse
   c) Sheep
   d) Mare

97. In which type of implantation does the blastocyst penetrate the uterine epithelium?
   a) Centric
   b) Interstitial
   c) Eccentric
   d) Artiodactyl

98. Which type of implantation occurs at a predetermined site such as the endometrial caruncle?
   a) Interstitial
   b) Centric
   c) Artiodactyl
   d) Eccentric

99. Which process involves the invagination of pluripotent cells and the formation of three germ layers?
   a) Organogenesis b) Gastrulation
   c) Implantation d) Differentiation

100. The primitive streak is formed by the migration of cells from which part of the germ disc?
   a) Cephalic end b) Caudal end
   c) Peripheral margin d) Central part

101. What does the notochord eventually become in the vertebral column?
   a) Nucleus pulposus of intervertebral discs
   b) Vertebrae
   c) Endoderm
   d) Amniotic cavity

102. Which mesodermal layer forms the vertebrae, ribs, and scapula?
   a) Myotome b) Sclerotome
   c) Dermatome d) Intermediate mesoderm

103. Which somite derivative forms the musculature for its own segment?
   a) Sclerotome b) Dermatome
   c) Myotome d) Paraxial mesoderm

104. At which stage do somites first begin to appear in the chick embryo?
   a) 21 hours of incubation b) 24 hours of incubation
   c) 27 hours of incubation d) 33 hours of incubation

105. In mammals, what is the maximum number of somite pairs present?
   a) 30 pairs b) 40 pairs
   c) 44 pairs d) 50 pairs

106. The somites give rise to which of the following structures?
   a) Heart and blood vessels
   b) Gut and respiratory lining
   c) Skeletal muscle, vertebrae, and dermis
   d) Nervous system and glands

107. Which layer forms the epidermis, hair, and nails?
   a) Mesoderm b) Endoderm
   c) Ectoderm d) Neural plate

108. What does the mesoderm give rise to?
   a) Nervous system
   b) Epidermis
   c) Skeletal tissue, muscles, and blood vascular system
   d) Gut lining

109. Which structure is formed from the endoderm's foregut?
   a) Liver and pancreas
   b) Mucous membrane of the alimentary tract
   c) Urinary bladder
   d) Prostate gland

110. From which germ layer do the gonads and adrenal cortex originate?
   a) Ectoderm b) Endoderm
   c) Mesoderm d) Neural plate

111. The epithelial lining of the respiratory system is derived from which germ layer?
   a) Ectoderm b) Endoderm
   c) Mesoderm d) Neural plate

112. The sclerotome from somites contributes to which body structure?
   a) Skin b) Muscles
   c) Vertebrae d) Nervous system

113. Which of the following is a derivative of the dermatome?
   a) Vertebrae b) Muscle tissue
   c) Dermis and subcutaneous tissue d) Nervous system

114. The coelom is formed by the splitting of which layer?
   a) Ectoderm b) Endoderm
   c) Mesoderm d) Neural plate

115. In which area is mesenchyme most commonly found?
   a) Skin
   b) Lining of the digestive tract
   c) Beneath the epithelium and within connective tissue
   d) Nervous system

116. The lateral mesoderm differentiates into which of the following?
   a) Heart and blood vessels b) Epidermis
   c) Neural tube d) Digestive system lining

117. Which mesodermal derivative forms the mesenteries of the gut?
   a) Somatic mesoderm b) Splanchnic mesoderm
   c) Intermediate mesoderm d) Paraxial mesoderm

118. The mesoderm surrounding the somites forms which of the following structures?
   a) Muscles of the limbs b) Derivatives of the skin
   c) Cartilage and bone d) Urogenital organs

119. The development of the urogenital system is primarily influenced by which mesodermal layer?
   a) Lateral mesoderm b) Paraxial mesoderm
   c) Intermediate mesoderm d) Splanchnic mesoderm

120. The notochord induces the formation of which embryonic structure?
   a) Neural tube
   b) Somites
   c) Gut
   d) Limb buds

121. Which embryonic structure is primarily involved in nutrient and gas exchange between the mother and fetus?
   a) Amnion
   b) Chorion
   c) Allantois
   d) Yolk sac

122. The placenta is derived from which two tissues?
   a) Maternal endometrium and embryonic chorion
   b) Amnion and yolk sac
   c) Mesoderm and ectoderm
   d) Ectoderm and endoderm

123. Which structure provides cushioning and protection to the developing embryo?
   a) Yolk sac
   b) Amniotic sac
   c) Placenta
   d) Chorion

124. What is the primary function of the yolk sac in human embryos?
   a) Blood cell formation in early development
   b) Gas exchange
   c) Protection of the embryo
   d) Nourishment of the embryo

125. The process of forming the neural tube from the neural plate is known as:
   a) Organogenesis
   b) Neurulation
   c) Gastrulation
   d) Somite formation

126. Which of the following animals shows a discoidal type of implantation?
   a) Human
   b) Mouse
   c) Cow
   d) Horse

127. Which type of implantation is seen in the mare and pig?
   a) Discoidal
   b) Cotyledonary
   c) Zonary
   d) Centric

128. Which type of implantation is observed in ruminants?
   a) Discoidal
   b) Cotyledonary
   c) Zonary
   d) Interstitial

129. Which animal is characterized by zonary implantation?
   a) Dog
   b) Horse
   c) Cow
   d) Cat

130. In which type of implantation does the blastocyst invade deeply into the uterine wall?
   a) Interstitial
   b) Eccentric
   c) Cotyledonary
   d) Zonary

131. In which type of placenta are chorionic villi scattered over the entire surface of the chorion?

a) Cotyledonary
b) Discoid
c) Zonary
d) Diffuse

132. Which structure in the umbilical cord carries impure blood from the fetus to the placenta?

a) Umbilical Vein
b) Umbilical Artery
c) Ductus Venosus
d) Foramen Ovale

133. Which type of placenta is characterized by the maternal endothelium and chorionic villi being directly in contact?

a) Syndesmo-chorial
b) Endothelio-chorial
c) Epithelio-chorial
d) Haemo-chorial

134. What does the ductus venosus do in fetal circulation?

a) Connects the right and left atria
b) Bypasses the hepatic circulation and connects the umbilical vein to the posterior vena cava
c) Carries oxygenated blood from the placenta to the fetus
d) Connects the pulmonary artery to the aorta

135. Which type of placenta is present in humans and has a villous structure with a thick layer of maternal tissue separating the fetal and maternal blood?

a) Haemo-chorial
b) Endothelio-chorial
c) Epithelio-chorial
d) Syndesmo-chorial

136. Which membrane contributes to the formation of the umbilical cord in mammals?

a) Yolk Sac
b) Chorion
c) Amnion
d) Allantois

137. What is the primary role of the amniotic fluid during fetal development?

a) Provides nutrients
b) Facilitates fetal movement
c) Protects the fetus from injury and maintains a stable temperature
d) Assists in respiratory function

138. In which type of placenta do the chorionic villi form a series of discrete cotyledons, each of which is surrounded by maternal tissue?

a) Cotyledonary
b) Discoid
c) Diffuse
d) Zonary

139. Which part of the fetal circulation system allows blood to bypass the non-functional fetal lungs?

a) Foramen Ovale
b) Ductus Arteriosus
c) Ductus Venosus
d) Umbilical Arteries

140. Which of the following structures helps in removing metabolic wastes from the fetal blood?
   a) Umbilical Vein
   b) Umbilical Artery
   c) Allantois
   d) Yolk Sac

141. Which fetal structure is responsible for the direct transport of oxygenated blood from the placenta to the fetal heart?
   a) Umbilical Vein
   b) Umbilical Artery
   c) Ductus Arteriosus
   d) Foramen Ovale

142. Which of the following best describes the function of the yolk sac in embryonic development?
   a) Provides nutrients to the embryo
   b) Acts as a respiratory surface
   c) Produces blood cells in early development
   d) Protects the embryo from physical damage

143. Which embryonic membrane is responsible for forming the outermost protective layer around the embryo?
   a) Amnion
   b) Chorion
   c) Yolk Sac
   d) Allantois

144. What structure allows for the exchange of gases and nutrients between the mother and fetus?
   a) Umbilical Cord
   b) Amniotic Sac
   c) Placenta
   d) Yolk Sac

145. Which embryonic membrane forms the primary site of exchange of nutrients and waste products in avian species?
   a) Amnion
   b) Yolk Sac
   c) Allantois
   d) Chorion

146. What is the primary function of the amniotic sac?
   a) Nourish the embryo
   b) Facilitate gas exchange
   c) Protect the embryo from mechanical shock
   d) Produce hormones

147. Which fetal structure helps to drain blood from the placenta to the fetal liver?
   a) Umbilical Vein
   b) Umbilical Artery
   c) Ductus Venosus
   d) Foramen Ovale

148. What is the main function of the chorionic villi in the placenta?
   a) To absorb nutrients
   b) To facilitate maternal-fetal gas exchange
   c) To produce hormones
   d) To protect the fetus

149. Which fetal structure connects the left and right atria of the heart, allowing blood to bypass the lungs?

a) Foramen Ovale
b) Ductus Arteriosus
c) Ductus Venosus
d) Umbilical Vein

Answer Key

1	c	2	b	3	b	4	a	5	a	6	d	7	b
8	c	9	c	10	c	11	c	12	b	13	b	14	a
15	d	16	c	17	a	18	c	19	c	20	b	21	c
22	a	23	d	24	c	25	b	26	c	27	c	28	c
29	c	30	a	31	a	32	b	33	a	34	a	35	b
36	b	37	b	38	a	39	c	40	a	41	a	42	c
43	a	44	d	45	a	46	b	47	b	48	b	49	c
50	b	51	a	52	b	53	b	54	b	55	c	56	c
57	b	58	d	59	a	60	a	61	b	62	b	63	b
64	b	65	b	66	a	67	b	68	b	69	a	70	b
71	b	72	a	73	b	74	c	75	d	76	b	77	a
78	b	79	b	80	a	81	c	82	b	83	a	84	a
85	a	86	b	87	c	88	b	89	a	90	b	91	d
92	a	93	b	94	b	95	b	96	b	97	b	98	c
99	b	100	b	101	a	102	b	103	c	104	a	105	c
106	c	107	c	108	c	109	a	110	c	111	b	112	c
113	c	114	c	115	c	116	a	117	b	118	c	119	c
120	a	121	b	122	a	123	b	124	a	125	b	126	a
127	d	128	b	129	d	130	a	131	d	132	b	133	b
134	b	135	a	136	d	137	c	138	a	139	b	140	c
141	a	142	c	143	b	144	c	145	b	146	c	147	c
148	b	149	b										

2

Genetic, Chromosomal and Environmental Factors Affecting Prenatal Development

Divya Gupta, Rajesh Rajput, Virender Pathak and Parul Shukla

Department of Veterinary Anatomy, DGCN COVAS, CSKHPKV, Palampur-176062

Introduction

Prenatal development is a crucial phase in the life of an organism during which the foundation for its future health and survival is established. In animals, the prenatal development is influenced by a complex interaction of genetic, chromosomal and environmental factors. These factors play a pivotal role in determining the phenotype, viability and overall health of the developing organism.

The abnormalities of the structure or function of cells, tissues or organs present at birth are termed as congenital defects. These developmental defects can be caused by genetic, chromosomal and environmental factors.

A. Genetic Factors

Genes are the fundamental units of inheritance and their expression controls the development and functioning of all living organisms. In prenatal development, genetic factors provide the blueprint on which the formation and differentiation of tissues and organs is depend. These factors influence a range of developmental processes which include the timing and coordination of cell division and the development of specific structures.`

1. **Gene Expression and Regulation:** Proper gene expression and regulation are essential for normal prenatal development. Genes are activated or suppressed at specific times during development and the precise regulation of these genes ensures the correct formation of tissues and organs. The mutations in key developmental genes can lead to malformations or developmental disorders.
2. **Inherited Traits and Developmental Variation:** Inherited genetic traits can influence the rate of prenatal development and the eventual size and characteristics of the offspring. For example, certain breeds of animals have genetic predispositions for faster growth rates, larger body sizes or distinct physical features which are evident even during prenatal development. Selective breeding practices in domesticated animals often aim to enhance these traits but they can also accidently introduce genetic disorders or vulnerabilities.
3. **Epigenetic Modifications:** Epigenetic factors such as DNA methylation and histone modifications also plays a crucial role in regulating gene expression during

prenatal development. These modifications can be influenced by environmental factors and they can have long-lasting effects on the phenotype of the organism. Epigenetic changes can be passed on to future generations even though they do not involve alterations to the DNA sequence itself. This highlights the importance of both genetic and environmental factors in shaping prenatal development.

B. Chromosomal Factors

Chromosomal factors refer to the structure and number of chromosomes within the cells of the developing organism. Any abnormalities in chromosome number or structure can have significant effects on prenatal development often leading to developmental disorders or pregnancy loss.

1. **Chromosomal Abnormalities:** Chromosomal abnormalities such as aneuploidy (the presence of an abnormal number of chromosomes) are a major cause of developmental disorders and early embryonic mortality. The conditions such as monosomy (missing a chromosome) or trisomy (having an extra chromosome) can lead to severe developmental issues. For example, trisomy 21 leads to Down syndrome, a condition associated with developmental delays and physical abnormalities. In animals, similar chromosomal anomalies can result in deformities or non-viable offspring.
2. **Structural Chromosomal Defects:** Structural defects in chromosomes such as deletions, duplications, inversions and translocations can disrupt normal prenatal development. These defects can interfere with the normal function of essential genes leading to developmental delays, malformations or even embryonic lethality. Chromosomal rea rrangements can also affect fertility as they can lead to improper segregation of chromosomes during cell division which results in the production of non-viable gametes.

C. Environmental Factors

The environment in which prenatal development occurs can have a profound impact on the health and development of the offspring. Environmental factors include both the external environment (e.g. temperature, nutrition, toxins) and the internal environment of the mother's body (e.g. hormone levels, uterine conditions). These factors can interact with genetic and chromosomal influences too.

1. **Maternal Nutrition:** Maternal nutrition is one of the most important environmental factors affecting prenatal development. A deficiency in key nutrients such as vitamins, minerals or proteins can lead to developmental delays, birth defects or even miscarriage. For example, a deficiency in folic acid is associated with neural tube defects in animals. Also excessive nutrient intake particularly of certain vitamins or minerals can also have detrimental effects on prenatal development.
2. **Toxins and Teratogens:** Teratogens are substances that can cause malformations or developmental abnormalities in the developing embryo or foetus. These can include environmental toxins e.g. pesticides, heavy metals, drugs and certain infections. Exposure to teratogens during critical periods of prenatal development can lead to congenital abnormalities such as limb malformations, heart defects or brain damage. The severity of the effect depends on the timing, duration and dose of the exposure.

3. **Temperature and Climate:** Temperature and climate conditions can influence prenatal development in animals, particularly in species that rely on external temperatures for incubation such as reptiles and some birds. Extreme temperatures can disrupt normal developmental processes which leads to abnormalities or developmental delays. For example, temperature fluctuations during egg incubation in birds can affect the growth and survival of the embryo. In mammals, maternal body temperature can also influence prenatal development as fever or hyperthermia during pregnancy can increase the risk of neural tube defects.
4. **Hormonal Influences:** Hormonal imbalances in the mother can have significant effects on prenatal development. For example, abnormal levels of hormones such as oestrogen, progesterone or cortisol can disrupt the normal growth and differentiation of tissues and organs in the developing embryo. Stress during pregnancy also elevates maternal cortisol levels which affect the development of the offspring's brain and behaviour in some animal species.
5. **Intrauterine Environment:** The intrauterine environment includes the quality of the placenta and the availability of oxygen and nutrients which plays a critical role in prenatal development. Poor placental function can result in restricted foetal growth or hypoxia which can have long-term consequences for the health and development of the offspring. Conditions such as preeclampsia or gestational diabetes in the mother can also adversely affect the intrauterine environment leading to complications in prenatal development.

Prenatal development in animals is a highly complex and dynamic process influenced by genetic, chromosomal and environmental factors. Each of these factors plays a unique role in shaping the developmental pathway of the organism. Disruptions in any of these areas can lead to significant developmental challenges. Genetic factors provide the plan for development, while chromosomal integrity ensures proper cell division and differentiation. Environmental factors both external and internal can modify the expression of genetic information and directly affect the health and viability of the developing organism.

Multiple Choice Questions

1. What is a congenital defect?
   a) A defect acquired after birth
   b) A defect presents at birth
   c) A temporary condition that resolves over time
   d) A defect caused by external factors after birth
2. Congenital defects are typically caused by:
   a) Genetic factors
   b) Environmental factors
   c) Unknown factors
   d) All of the above
3. Can congenital defects be detected before birth?
   a) No, they can only be diagnosed after birth
   b) Yes, some can be detected through prenatal screening and tests
   c) Yes, all congenital defects can be detected before birth
   d) It depends on the defect's severity

4. Which of the following is NOT a characteristic of congenital defects?
   a) They are present at birth
   b) They are always life-threatening
   c) They can vary in severity
   d) They can affect different parts of the body
5. Which of the following best describes a mutation?
   a) A natural, beneficial change in an organism
   b) A change in the DNA sequence of an organism
   c) A harmful alteration in protein structure
   d) A temporary change in an organism's behaviour
6. Which enzyme is responsible for correcting errors in DNA replication?
   a) DNA ligase
   b) DNA polymerase
   c) Helicase
   d) RNA polymerase
7. Which of the following can cause mutations in DNA?
   a) UV radiation
   b) Chemicals
   c) Viruses
   d) All of the above
8. A mutation in which a segment of DNA is copied and inserted into the genome is called:
   a) Deletion
   b) Insertion
   c) Duplication
   d) Inversion
9. What is a mutagen?
   a) A mutation that benefits the organism
   b) An agent that causes a change in DNA
   c) A protein that repairs DNA
   d) A genetic sequence without mutations
10. What is a chromosomal abnormality?
   a) A mutation in a single gene
   b) An alteration in the number or structure of chromosomes
   c) A defect in the cell membrane
   d) A disorder caused by environmental factors
11. Which chromosomal abnormality is characterized by an extra copy of chromosome 21?
   a) Turner syndrome
   b) Klinefelter syndrome
   c) Down syndrome
   d) Patau syndrome
12. Which chromosomal condition involves a female having only one X chromosome?
   a) Turner syndrome
   b) Klinefelter syndrome
   c) Jacobs syndrome
   d) Triple X syndrome
13. Patau syndrome is caused by an extra chromosome in which pair?
   a) 13
   b) 18
   c) 21
   d) X

14. Which of the following is a sex chromosome abnormality?
    a) Trisomy 13
    b) Trisomy 18
    c) Turner syndrome
    d) Down syndrome
15. Which syndrome is caused by a deletion on the short arm of chromosome 5?
    a) Cri-du-chat syndrome
    b) Angelman syndrome
    c) Prader-Willi syndrome
    d) Williams syndrome
16. What is a teratogen?
    a) A substance that promotes cell growth
    b) A substance that causes birth defects
    c) A substance that enhances immune function
    d) A substance that prevents infections
17. Which of the following is a known teratogen?
    a) Folic acid
    b) Vitamin A
    c) Vitamin C
    d) Glucose
18. During which stage of pregnancy are teratogens most harmful?
    a) First trimester
    b) Second trimester
    c) Third trimester
    d) Postnatal
19. Teratogens can cause malformations through interference with which of the following processes?
    a) Cell division
    b) Hormone regulation
    c) Gene expressions.
    d) All of the above
20. Which of the following animals is most commonly affected by DDT contamination?
    a) Fish
    b) Cattle
    c) Birds
    d) Amphibians
21. What is the primary way DDT enters the food chain in animals?
    a) Inhalation
    b) Ingestion of contaminated water
    c) Skin absorption
    d) Consumption of contaminated food
22. DDT primarily accumulates in which part of an animal's body?
    a) Muscle tissue
    b) Bones
    c) Liver
    d) Fatty tissue
23. Which reproductive issue is commonly associated with DDT contamination in birds?
    a) Eggshell thinning
    b) Decreased fertility
    c) Increased hatching success
    d) Premature molting

24. A metabolic bi product of DDT known as DDE exert its effect on animals by:
    a) Mimicking estrogen activity
    b) Inhibiting the effectiveness of androgens
    c) Both a & b
    d) By mimicking insulin activity
25. The damaging effect of DDT on wildlife species was reported in early:
    a) 1980s b) 1970s
    c) 1960s d) 1950s
26. Dioxin toxicity primarily affects which system in animals?
    a) Respiratory system b) Cardiovascular system
    c) Immune and endocrine systems d) Digestive system
27. What is the main route of dioxin exposure in animals?
    a) Inhalation b) Skin absorption
    c) Ingestion of contaminated feed d) Direct Injection
28. Which species is most sensitive to dioxin toxicity?
    a) Chickens b) Fish
    c) Cattle d) Rats
29. What are the common symptoms of dioxin toxicity in animals?
    a) Fever and lethargy
    b) Skin lesions, reproductive failure and immunosuppression
    c) Weight gain
    d) None of the above
30. Which of the following method is commonly used to reduce dioxin exposure in animals?
    a) Increased antibiotic usage
    b) Improved feed quality and source control
    c) Reducing water intake
    d) Prolonged sunlight exposure
31. Which of the following is a known teratogenic effect of lead exposure during pregnancy?
    a) Neural tube defects b) Cleft palate
    c) Limb deformities d) All of the above
32. Lead exposure during pregnancy primarily affects which system in the developing foetus?
    a) Digestive system b) Nervous system
    c) Muscular system d) Respiratory system
33. Which organ in the foetus is most vulnerable to the teratogenic effects of lead?
    a) Liver b) Brain
    c) Heart d) Lungs

34. Polychlorinated biphenyls have been shown to cause what kind of reproductive effects in wildlife?
    a) Infertility
    b) Increased litter size
    c) Enhanced reproductive success
    d) Early weaning of offspring
35. Polychlorinated biphenyls interfere with which system in the body to cause teratogenic effects?
    a) Nervous system
    b) Endocrine system
    c) Respiratory system
    d) Immune system
36. Which virus is known to cause cerebellar hypoplasia in calves?
    a) Foot-and-mouth disease virus
    b) Bovine viral diarrhoea virus (BVDV)
    c) Parvovirus
    d) Rabies virus
37. What is the primary teratogenic effect of the bluetongue virus in sheep?
    a) Limb deformities
    b) Hydranencephaly
    c) Cataracts
    d) Cardiac defects
38. Which virus can cause abortion and fetal mummification in pigs?
    a) Porcine reproductive and respiratory syndrome virus (PRRSV)
    b) Foot-and-mouth disease virus
    c) Classical swine fever virus
    d) Influenza virus
39. Which bacteria can cross the placenta and cause abortion or stillbirth in ruminants?
    a) Mycoplasma
    b) Listeria monocytogenes
    c) Staphylococcus aureus
    d) Bacillus anthracis
40. Which protozoan can cause fetal malformations and abortion in sheep?
    a) Giardia
    b) Neospora caninum
    c) Toxoplasma gondii
    d) Cryptosporidium
41. Which bacterial agent is known to cause abortion in cattle, swine, and sheep?
    a) Brucella spp.
    b) Streptococcus spp.
    c) Pasteurella spp.
    d) Clostridium spp.
42. The primary teratogenic effect of Rift Valley fever virus in ruminants is:
    a) Blindness
    b) Musculoskeletal deformities
    c) Encephalopathy
    d) Abortion and stillbirth
43. Which virus can cause fetal resorption and mummification in dogs?
    a) Canine distemper virus
    b) Canine herpesvirus
    c) Parvovirus
    d) Rabies virus
44. Which protozoan causes abortion and stillbirth in cattle and is transmitted through the faeces of infected dogs?
    a) Toxoplasma gondii
    b) Eimeria spp.
    c) Neospora caninum
    d) Sarcocystis spp.

45. Which of the following viruses can lead to skeletal deformities in pigs?
    a) African swine fever virus b) Classical swine fever virus
    c) Swine vesicular disease virus d) PRRS virus

46. What teratogenic effect is most commonly associated with rubella virus in humans, which can be compared to similar effects in animals?
    a) Heart defects b) Blindness
    c) Deafness d) All of the above

47. Congenital goitre is caused by:
    a) Folic acid b) Vitamin A
    c) Radioactive Iodine d) Aflatoxin

48. Which mineral deficiency causes the increase in neonatal mortality and goitre in domestic animals:
    a) Folic acid b) Vitamin A
    c) Iodine d) Aflatoxin

49. Which mineral deficiency in pregnant ewes leads to defective fetal myelination which leads to swayback condition in neonate at the time of birth?
    a) Copper b) Selenium
    c) Iron d) Calcium

50. Which Vitamin deficiency in pregnant sow leads to ocular agenesis in piglets born?
    a) Vitamin A b) Vitamin B
    c) Vitamin C d) Vitamin D

51. Congenital blindness in calves is caused by:
    a) Deficiency of vitamin A b) Excess of vitamin A
    c) Deficiency of vitamin D d) Excess of vitamin D

52. Which of these mycotoxins cause teratogenic effect?
    a) Aflatoxin b) Patulin
    c) Both a & b d) None of the above

53. Which mycotoxin mimics oestrogenic activity and can cause foetal malformations when fed to pregnant animals?
    a) Aflatoxin b) Zearalenone
    c) Patulin d) None of the above

54. Which of the following animals is most susceptible to teratogenic effects from zearalenone exposure?
    a) Cattle b) Pigs
    c) Chickens d) Horses

.55. In cattle, exposure to high levels of ergot alkaloids during pregnancy may result in:
    a) Limb deformities b) Abortion
    c) Kidney failure d) Heart defects

56. Mycotoxins can cause teratogenic effects in developing embryos by:
    a) Directly damaging DNA
    b) Inhibiting fetal cell growth
    c) Causing immune suppression
    d) All of the above

57. The severity of teratogenic effects caused by mycotoxins is dependent on:
    a) Dose and duration of exposure
    b) Age of the mother
    c) Breed of the animal
    d) Type of feed consumed

58. Which of the following best defines the teratogenic effect of hyperthermia?
    a) Abnormal cell division
    b) Developmental abnormalities in the fetus due to maternal overheating
    c) Excessive growth of fetal organs
    d) Premature birth due to dehydration in the mother

59. Which of the following conditions is a potential teratogenic outcome of maternal hyperthermia during pregnancy?
    a) Microcephaly
    b) Hypertension
    c) Autism
    d) Down syndrome

60. At what stage of pregnancy is the fetus most vulnerable to the teratogenic effects of hyperthermia?
    a) First trimester
    b) Second trimester
    c) Third trimester
    d) Fetal stage after birth

61. Which of the following best describes the teratogenic effects of ionizing radiation on developing animal embryos?
    a) Only affects adult animals
    b) Can cause birth defects, growth retardation, and malformations
    c) Primarily affects the nervous system of adult animals
    d) Causes no harm to the developing embryo

62. Which of the following is a common malformation observed in animals exposed to ionizing radiation during pregnancy?
    a) Polydactyly
    b) Microcephaly
    c) Color blindness
    d) Extra limbs

63. Which of the following factors influence the severity of teratogenic effects caused by ionizing radiation in animals?
    a) Dosage and stage of development
    b) Animal species and sunlight exposure
    c) Gender and diet of the mother
    d) Water intake and sleep patterns

64. Which of the following plants is known to cause severe congenital deformities in cattle when ingested during early pregnancy?
    a) Lupine
    b) Alfalfa
    c) Clover
    d) Barley

65. Veratrum californicum (Corn Lily) ingestion by pregnant sheep commonly leads to which congenital defect?
    a) Blindness
    b) Cyclopia (single eye defect)
    c) Short limbs
    d) Heart defects
66. Which toxic substance found in poison hemlock (Conium maculatum) primarily affects prenatal development in livestock?
    a) Cyanide
    b) Alkaloids
    c) Tannins
    d) Oxalates
67. Which compound is widely used anthelmintics in domestic animals can lead to skeletal and vascular anomalies in ovine embryo when it is administered in pregnant ewes?
    a) Benzimidazole
    b) Steroids
    c) Friseofulvin
    d) Methadone
68. What is the effect of administering corticosteroids during pregnancy in animals?
    a) Enhanced fetal growth
    b) Risk of fetal malformations
    c) Increased placental blood flow
    d) Prevention of fetal infections
69. Which drug, commonly used to treat bacterial infections, is linked to hearing loss in animal offspring if administered during pregnancy?
    a) Penicillin
    b) Gentamicin
    c) Amoxicillin
    d) Cephalexin
70. Which therapeutic drug is widely used as anthelmintic in sheep and when administered in pregnant ewes causes skeletal, renal and vascular anomalies in ovine embryos?
    a) Griseofulvim
    b) Tetracycline
    c) Bezimidazole compounds
    d) Coumarin derivatives
71. Which of the following is a major genetic factor affecting prenatal development in animals?
    a) Maternal nutrition
    b) Paternal age
    c) Inherited genetic mutations
    d) Environmental temperature
72. Maternal malnutrition during pregnancy can lead to which of the following in the offspring?
    a) Increased birth weight
    b) Congenital malformations
    c) Enhanced growth rate
    d) Stronger immunity
73. The gestational stage during which a fetus is most susceptible to teratogens is:
    a) The first trimester
    b) The second trimester
    c) The third trimester
    d) The final week of gestation
74. A lack of which vitamin during pregnancy is associated with neural tube defects in developing offspring?
    a) Vitamin A
    b) Vitamin D
    c) Vitamin K
    d) Folic acid

75. Which of the following conditions during pregnancy increases the risk of intrauterine growth restriction (IUGR) in animals?
    a) Overnutrition
    b) Maternal weight
    c) High protein intake
    d) Malnutrition

76. Prenatal exposure to high levels of glucocorticoids can result in:
    a) Faster fetal development
    b) Enhanced fetal immunity
    c) Fetal growth retardation
    d) Increased litter size

77. Which of the following factors during pregnancy can lead to premature birth?
    a) Overexertion
    b) Stress
    c) Both a and b
    d) None of the above

78. Which of the following nutrients is critical to preventing congenital skeletal deformities in developing fetuses?
    a) Vitamin C
    b) Vitamin K
    c) Calcium
    d) Vitamin B12

79. Which of the following can directly affect placental function and thus fetal development?
    a) Infectious diseases
    b) Maternal blood pressure
    c) Nutrient supply
    d) All of the above

80. Exposure to pesticides during pregnancy is classified under which factor affecting prenatal development?
    a) Genetic
    b) Environmental
    c) Mechanical
    d) Epigenetic

81. Which feature determine whether the congenital disease is caused by chromosomal factor or by teratogenic agents?
    a) Number of animals affected
    b) Geographical distribution
    c) Mechanism of disease production
    d) All of the above

82. Abnormalities of the structures or the function of cells, tissue or organs present at birth are termed as:
    a) Teratogenic effects
    b) Congenital defects
    c) Acquired defects
    d) Mutational effects

83. A structural defect which results from the destruction of a previously normal structure due to interruption of blood supply is refer to:
    a) Disruption
    b) Malformation
    c) Deformation
    d) All of the above

84. Which statement is not correct regarding congenital defects?
    a) Congenital defects can be caused by genetic factors and environmental influences.
    b) Congenital effects in lambs, calves and foals occurs to an upper limit of 3-4%.
    c) The aetiology of congenital defects can be always known.
    d) These defects are reported infrequently in cats.

85. Which method can be used to observe deletion or aberrations occurring at chromosomal level?
   a) Histology b) Cytology
   c) Enzymology d) None of the above

86. The Toxoplasma gondii is major cause of abortion which species?
   a) Equine b) Bovine

87. Which of the following factors has the most direct influence on the prenatal development of poultry?
   a) Age of the hen b) Temperature during incubation
   c) Egg size d) Light exposure during laying

88. Which of the following substances is considered a teratogen in animals?
   a) Vitamins b) Antibiotics
   c) Thalidomide d) Water

89. Which of the following is NOT a common type of teratogen?
   a) Radiation b) Nutritional deficiency
   c) Genetic mutation d) Infectious agents

90. Which vitamin deficiency is known to be a teratogen in animals?
   a) Vitamin C b) Vitamin D
   c) Folic acid d) Vitamin B12

91. The use of corticosteroids during pregnancy in animals can cause which congenital abnormality?
   a) Limb deformities b) Heart defects
   c) Cleft palate d) All of the above

92. Which of the following livestock is most susceptible to teratogenic effects of viral infections?
   a) Cattle b) Sheep
   c) Pigs d) Chickens

93. Which of the following chemicals is a well-known teratogen in farm animals?
   a) Pesticides b) Herbicides
   c) Lead d) All of the above

94. Brucella spp. is a teratogen primarily affecting which organ system?
   a) Cardiovascular system b) Nervous system
   c) Reproductive system d) Respiratory system

95. Which mineral overdose can act as a teratogen in livestock?
   a) Zinc b) Selenium
   c) Copper d) Manganese

96. Which of the following conditions results from incomplete fusion of the neural tube during development?
   a) Spina bifida b) Hydrocephalus
   c) Umbilical hernia d) Cryptorchidism

97. Which of the following congenital defects is characterized by the absence of a limb or part of a limb?
    a) Amelia
    b) Arthrogryposis
    c) Syndactyly
    d) Achondroplasia
98. Which nutrient deficiency in pregnant animals can lead to skeletal abnormalities in offspring?
    a) Vitamin D
    b) Vitamin B12
    c) Vitamin E
    d) Vitamin C
99. Which virus is known to cause prenatal defects in pigs, including stillbirths and mummified foetuses?
    a) Bovine herpesvirus
    b) Porcine parvovirus
    c) Canine distemper virus
    d) Rabies virus
100. Which of the following parameters can determine the probable aetiology of congenital defects observed in a group of pregnant animals?
    a) Species
    b) Number of animals
    c) Nature of congenital malformations
    d) All of the above

Answer Key

1	b	2	d	3	b	4	b	5	b	6	b	7	d
8	c	9	b	10	b	11	c	12	a	13	a	14	c
15	a	16	b	17	b	18	a	19	d	20	c	21	d
22	d	23	a	24	c	25	c	26	c	27	c	28	b
29	b	30	b	31	d	32	b	33	b	34	a	35	b
36	b	37	b	38	a	39	b	40	c	41	a	42	d
43	b	44	c	45	b	46	d	47	c	48	c	49	a
50	a	51	b	52	c	53	b	54	b	55	b	56	d
57	a	58	b	59	a	60	a	61	b	62	b	63	a
64	a	65	b	66	b	67	a	68	b	69	b	70	c
71	c	72	b	73	a	74	d	75	d	76	c	77	c
78	c	79	d	80	b	81	d	82	b	83	a	84	c
85	b	86	b	87	b	88	c	89	c	90	c	91	d
92	b	93	d	94	c	95	b	96	a	97	a	98	a
99	c	100	d										

3

Cell Division
Growth and Differentiation

Manoj Kumar Sinha, Avnish Kumar Gautam, G.D Singh, Anil Kumar Safi and Manju Sinha

Department Veterinary Anatomy, Bihar Veterinary College, Patna, Bihar
Bihar Animal Sciences University, Patna, Bihar
Institute of Animal Health & Production, Patna, Bihar
Department of Animal and Fishery Resources, Bihar, Bihar

Introduction

It is a fundamental biological process in which one cell splits into two or more daughter cells. Both unicellular and multicellular organisms rely heavily on it for growth, development, repair, and reproduction. There are two main types of cell division: mitosis and meiosis. Mitosis occurs in somatic cells and produces two genetically identical daughter cells that share the same chromosomal number as the parent cell. This process is necessary for tissue development and repair. Meiosis, on the other hand, happens in germ cells and results in the formation of gametes, which reduces the number of chromosomes by half to ensure genetic diversity in progeny. Proper regulation of cell division is vital for maintaining cellular health, and disruptions in this process can lead to disorders like cancer.

The different stages of cell division is as follows:-

1. Interphase

- Although not a component of mitosis, interphase is essential for preparing the cell for division. It is separated into three sub-phases:
- G1 phase (Gap 1): The cell expands in size while creating proteins and organelles. S phase (Synthesis): DNA replication occurs, guaranteeing that each daughter cell receives an identical copy of the genetic information.
- G2 phase (Gap 2): The cell continues to expand while new organelles are synthesised)

  The cell checks for DNA replication mistakes and gets ready for mitosis.

2. Prophase

- In this phase chromatin condenses into visible chromosomes, each made up of two sister chromatids linked at the centromere.
- The nuclear membrane breaks down, allowing the spindle fibres to interact with the chromosomes.

- The centrioles, which are little cylindrical structures in animal cells, begin to travel to opposing poles of the cell, and spindle fibres (made up of microtubules) form between them. These spindle fibres play an important role in guiding chromosomal movements.

3. Metaphase

- The spindle fibres are fully developed, and the chromosomes align along the metaphase plate.
- The centromeres of each chromosome connect it to spindle fibres at opposite poles. This assures that when the sister chromatids are split, they will migrate to different ends of the cell.
- Metaphase is an important checkpoint in mitosis because the cell ensures that all chromosomes are properly aligned and linked to the spindle apparatus before progressing.

4. Anaphase

- In anaphase spindle fibres pull the sister chromatids apart, causing each chromatid to go in the direction of the cell's opposite pole.
- The spindle fibres connected to the centromeres are getting shorter, which is what causes this separation. Once the chromatids are split, each is considered an independent chromosome.
- This phase makes sure that every daughter cell inherits the same set of chromosomes.

5. Telophase

- In this phase the chromosomes become less visible under a microscope when they decondense back into chromatin as they approach the poles of the cell.
- Each set of chromosomes at the poles is surrounded by a fresh nuclear membrane, resulting in the formation of two separate nuclei.
- As the spindle fibres disintegrate, the cell gets ready for the cytoplasm's ultimate separation.

6. Cytokinesis

- The division of the cytoplasm, known as cytokinesis, takes place either right after or concurrently with telophase.
- A cleavage furrow appears in animal cells, pinching the cell membrane inward until the cell divides into two separate daughter cells.
- A cell plate develops down the middle of plant cells. Eventually, a new cell wall that divides the two daughter cells forms from this plate.

The outcome of mitosis

- Two daughter cells that are genetically identical are produced with the completion of mitosis and cytokinesis.
- Each cell is prepared for interphase, where it can grow and eventually divide again if necessary.
- It has the same number of chromosomes as the original parent cell. In multicellular organisms, this mechanism is essential for growth, repair, and asexual reproduction.

Cell growth

It is an important process that involves increasing cell size and accumulating cellular components necessary for cell function. It takes place during the interphase of the cell cycle, namely in the G1 phase, when the cell produces proteins, lipids, and other macromolecules required for its structure and metabolism. This expansion is required to prepare the cell for division, ensuring that there are enough resources to form two viable daughter cells. A variety of factors drive cell growth, including nutrient availability, growth signals, and environmental circumstances. Growth factors, like hormones and cytokines, play a key role in signaling cells to grow and divide, coordinating overall tissue and organ development.

Cell differentiation

It is the process by which unspecialised cells, such as stem cells, transform into specialised cells with unique structures and functions. This process is critical for the formation of multicellular creatures because it allows cells to form tissues and organs, each with a distinct function, such as muscle cells, nerve cells, and blood cells. Gene expression variations cause differentiation, which are regulated by transcription factors and external cues from the cell's environment. When a cell divides, it often takes on a distinct shape, structure, and set of functions that it will keep for the rest of its existence. While most cells specialise through differentiation, some, such as stem cells, maintain the ability to differentiate into several cell types.

Multiple Choice Questions

1. What is cell differentiation?
   a) Cells growing larger
   b) Cells becoming specialized in structure and function
   c) Cells dividing rapidly
   d) Cells losing their nucleus
2. Which of the following is a primary result of cell differentiation?
   a) Genetic mutations
   b) Development of tissues and organs
   c) Uncontrolled cell growth
   d) Apoptosis
3. Which type of stem cells can differentiate into any cell type?
   a) Multipotent b) Unipotent
   c) Pluripotent d) Progenitor cells
4. What is the role of transcription factors in cell differentiation?
   a) They speed up cell division
   b) They guide gene expression for specialization
   c) They regulate cell growth
   d) They remove damaged DNA
5. What is the result of improper cell differentiation?
   a) Normal tissue formation
   b) Developmental disorders or diseases

c) Increased apoptosis
d) Enhanced immune response

6. In plants, cell differentiation occurs in which regions?
a) Leaves b) Stems
c) Roots d) Meristems

7. The spindle apparatus is formed during the ________ phase of mitosis.
a) Telophase b) Metaphase
c) Prophase d) Anaphase

8. Cyclin is associated with __________
a) Leptospirosis b) Glycolysis
c) Cylosis d) Mitosis

9. What is the primary role of cell growth in multicellular organisms?
a) Reproduction b) Energy production
c) Tissue repair and development d) Waste removal

10. Which of the following processes occurs during interphase?
a) Chromosomes condense b) DNA replication
c) Chromosome alignment d) Sister chromatid separation

11. At which stage of meiosis do homologous chromosomes separate?
a) Prophase I b) Metaphase I
c) Anaphase I d) Telophase I

12. How many chromosomes are present in each human gamete after meiosis?
a) 23 b) 46
c) 69 d) 92

13. What is the name of the checkpoints that control cell growth in the cell cycle?
a) Mitotic checkpoints b) Growth regulators
c) Cell cycle checkpoints d) Cytokinesis checkpoints

14. Which protein plays a key role in regulating cell growth and the cell cycle?
a) Actin b) Cyclin
c) Tubulin d) Keratin

15. _________ is a form of cell division which results in the creation of gametes or sex cells.
a) Mitosis b) Meiosis
c) Miosis d) None of the above

16. _____ is the number of DNA in the chromosome at the G2 stage of the cell cycle
a) 1 b) 2
c) 3 d) 0

17. Which of the following is NOT a factor that can inhibit cell growth?
a) Contact inhibition b) Nutrient scarcity
c) Growth factors d) DNA damage

18. In which part of the cell cycle does the cell spend the most time?
    a) G1 phase
    b) S phase
    c) G2 phase
    d) M phase
19. The longest stage in the cell cycle is
    a) Interphase
    b) Anaphase
    c) Metaphase
    d) None of the above
20. The _______ state implies the exit of cells from the cell cycle
    a) S
    b) G1
    c) G2
    d) G0
21. Excessive and uncontrolled cell growth is associated with which condition?
    a) Cancer
    b) Infection
    c) Muscle atrophy
    d) Diabetes
22. Which of the following nutrients is essential for cell growth?
    a) Oxygen
    b) Glucose
    c) Nitrogen
    d) Sodium chloride
23. Which process ensures that cells do not grow too large to maintain proper function?
    a) Cell division
    b) DNA replication
    c) Apoptosis
    d) Cell differentiation
24. At what stage in development does cell differentiation typically begin?
    a) Adult stage
    b) Blastocyst stage
    c) Embryonic stage
    d) Fetal stage
25. Which of the following factors influences cell differentiation?
    a) Gene expression
    b) DNA replication
    c) Chromosome number
    d) Cytokinesis
26. What are stem cells?
    a) Cells that have undergone differentiation
    b) Cells that are undifferentiated and can become specialized
    c) Cells that have stopped dividing
    d) Cells that are specialized for specific functions
27. Which of the following is responsible for promoting cell growth in animals?
    a) Growth hormone
    b) Insulin
    c) Glucagon
    d) Cortisol
28. Which of the following is a characteristic of a fully differentiated cell?
    a) It can still divide and become another cell type
    b) It has a specific structure and function
    c) It can revert back to an undifferentiated state
    d) It undergoes rapid division

29. What is the process called when a differentiated cell changes to another type of specialized cell?
    a) Redifferentiation
    b) Transdifferentiation
    c) Dedifferentiation
    d) Apoptosis
30. Which of the following tissues contain undifferentiated cells in adults?
    a) Liver
    b) Bone marrow
    c) Skin
    d) All of the above
31. What is hypertrophy in terms of cell growth?
    a) Increase in the number of cells
    b) Increase in the size of cells
    c) Decrease in cell number
    d) Division of cells
32. What happens if a cell cannot pass the G1 checkpoint?
    a) It proceeds to G2
    b) It undergoes apoptosis (programmed cell death)
    c) It goes into a resting state (G0)
    d) It directly enters mitosis
33. If an individual wants to view diakinesis, which of these would be
    a) Hair
    b) Leaf
    c) Onion root
    d) Flower bud
34. Chromosome structure can be observed best during ____
    a) Anaphase
    b) Metaphase
    c) Prophase
    d) None of the above
35. The term 'cell differentiation' refers to:
    a) Cells increasing in size
    b) Cells acquiring specialized functions
    c) Cells undergoing division
    d) Cells growing uncontrollably
36. Chromatids coiling in the meiotic and mitotic division is _____
    a) Plectonemic in both
    b) Paranemic in both
    c) Paranemic in mitosis and plectonemic in meiosis
    d) Plectonemic in mitosis and paranemic in meiosis
37. When there is an increase in the condensation of chromatin during the process of cell division –
    a) Heterochromatin increases
    b) Euchromatin increases
    c) Differentiation of euchromatin & heterochromatin decreases
    d) Differentiation of euchromatin & heterochromatin increases
38. Which of the following phases is part of mitosis?
    a) G1 phase
    b) S phase
    c) Prophase
    d) Cytokinesis

39. Which of the following factors directly affects cell growth?
    a) Oxygen levels b) Temperature
    c) Nutrient availability d) All of the above
40. Which phase of the cell cycle is primarily associated with cell growth?
    a) G1 phase b) G2 phase
    c) S phase d) M phase
41. During the G2 phase of the cell cycle, what primarily occurs?
    a) DNA replication
    b) Chromosome alignment
    c) Further cell growth and preparation for mitosis
    d) Cell division
42. During which phase of mitosis do the sister chromatids separate?
    a) Metaphase b) Anaphase
    c) Prophase d) Telophase
43. Which of the following is NOT a result of mitosis?
    a) Growth b) Repair
    c) Genetic variation d) Asexual reproduction.
44. Which of the following is an example of a differentiated cell?
    a) Zygote b) Muscle cell
    c) Stem cell d) Embryo
45. Which of the following types of stem cells are limited to differentiating into closely related cell types?
    a) Totipotent b) Multipotent
    c) Pluripotent d) Unipotent
46. What role does the environment play in cell differentiation?
    a) It has no effect
    b) It directly impacts gene expression and cell fate
    c) It limits the number of cell divisions
    d) It increases the rate of cell growth
47. What structure is responsible for organizing the spindle fibers during mitosis?
    a) Centriole b) Nucleus
    c) Ribosome d) Lysosome
48. In which phase of the cell cycle does DNA replication occur?
    a) G1 phase b) S phase
    c) G2 phase d) M phase
49. What is the main purpose of meiosis?
    a) To produce body cells b) To repair damaged cells
    c) To produce gametes d) To regulate the cell cycle

50. Synapsis is defined as the pairing of ________
    a) Acentric chromosomes
    b) Non-homologous chromosomes
    c) Any chromosomes
    d) Homologous chromosomes
51. Mitosis can be observed in ___
    a) Polyploid individual
    b) Diploid individual
    c) Haploid individual
    d) Both (1,) (2) and (3)
52. How many daughter cells are produced at the end of meiosis?
    a) 2
    b) 4
    c) 6
    d) 8
53. What is crossing over, and when does it occur?
    a) Exchange of DNA between sister chromatids, during prophase I
    b) Exchange of DNA between homologous chromosomes, during prophase I
    c) Fusion of two chromosomes, during metaphase I
    d) Separation of chromosomes, during anaphase II
54. The condensation of chromosomes is observed in ______
    a) Prophase 1
    b) Anaphase 1
    c) Metaphase 1
    d) None of the above
55. Nuclear DNA replicates in the ________ phase.
    a) G2 phase
    b) M phase
    c) S phase
    d) None of the above
56. Which of the following is a key difference between mitosis and meiosis?
    a) Mitosis produces genetically identical cells, while meiosis produces genetically diverse cells.
    b) Mitosis occurs only in reproductive cells, while meiosis occurs in body cells.
    c) Mitosis reduces the chromosome number by half, while meiosis maintains it.
    d) Mitosis involves two divisions, while meiosis involves one.
57. Which of the following is NOT a phase of mitosis?
    a) Prophase
    b) Metaphase
    c) Interphase
    d) Telophase
58. What is the name of the structure that forms during cytokinesis in animal cells?
    a) Cell plate
    b) Cleavage furrow
    c) Spindle fiber
    d) Centromere
59. Which of the following occurs during metaphase of mitosis?
    a) Chromosomes become visible under a microscope
    b) Chromosomes align at the equator of the cell
    c) Nuclear membrane reforms
    d) DNA replication occurs
60. __________ and _________ coined the term "Meiosis".
    a) Van Burin and Hertwig
    b) Boveri and Stuka
    c) Walleye and Hofmeister
    d) Farmer and Moore

61. The stage which serves as a connecting link between meiosis 1 and meiosis 2
    a) Interphase 2 b) Interphase 1
    c) Interkineses d) None of the above
62. The process of appearance of recombination nodules occurs at which sub-stage of prophase I in meiosis?
    a) Diakinesis b) Zygotene
    c) Pachytene d) Diplotene
63. Among eukaryotes, replication of DNA takes place in
    a) G2 Phase b) M phase
    c) S phase d) G1 phase
64. Which one of the following never occurs during mitotic cell division?
    a) Coiling and condensation chromatids
    b) Spindle fibers attach to Kinetochores of chromosomes
    c) Movement of centrioles toward opposite poles
    d) The pairing of homologous chromosomes
65. Regarding meiosis, which statement is incorrect?
    a) Four haploid cells form at the end of meiosis-II
    b) In meiosis, there are two stages: meiosis I and II
    c) DNA replication occurs in the S phase of meiosis-II
    d) The pairing of homologous and recombination chromosomes occurs during meiosis-1
66. When do the chromosomes pair during meiosis I?
    a) Leptotene b) Zygotene
    c) Pachytene d) Diplotene
67. What is true about the mitotic spindle?
    a) It is composed of actin and myosin microfilaments.
    b) It includes the kinetochore at the metaphase plate.
    c) It is composed of microtubules, which separate chromosomes at opposite poles of the cell.
    d) It originates only from centrioles of centrioles.
68. The synapsis occurs between
    a) male gamete and female gamete
    b) mRNA and ribosomes
    c) spindle fiber and centromere
    d) two homologous chromosomes
69. Which of the following precedes nuclear envelope reformation during the M phase of the cell cycle?
    a) Chromosome decondensation and reassembly of the nuclear lamina
    b) Transcription from chromosomes and nuclear leaf recombination
    c) Contraction ring formation and phragmoplast. formation
    d) Contraction ring formation and transcription from chromosomes.

70. What results in the formation of chiasmata?
    a) Exchange of parts of paired homologous chromosome
    b) Exchange of part of unpaired non-homologous chromosome
    c) Duplication of parts of paired homologous chromosome
    d) Loss of parts of unpaired non-homologous chromosome
71. The stage which serves as a connecting link between meiosis 1 and meiosis 2
    a) Interphase b) Interphase
    c) Interkinesis d) None of the above
72. ________ is the best stage to observe the shape, size, and number of chromosomes
    a) interphase b) metaphase
    c) prophase d) Telophase
73. If the Centromere is Located at the Proximity of the End of a Chromosome, It is Known as-
    a) Acrocentric b) Metacentric
    c) Telocentric d) Submetacentric
74. Which phase, out of the following phases, has most of the events occurring in it?
    a) G1 Phase b) G2 Phase
    c) M Phase d) Anaphase
75. Which of the following phases occupy 95% of the time involved in the cell cycle?
    a) Interphase b) Karyokinesis
    c) Metaphase d) Anaphase

Answer Key

1	b	2	b	3	c	4	b	5	b	6	d	7	b
8	d	9	c	10	b	11	c	12	a	13	c	14	b
15	b	16	b	17	b	18	a	19	a	20	d	21	a
22	b	23	a	24	c	25	a	26	b	27	a	28	b
29	b	30	d	31	b	32	c	33	d	34	b	35	b
36	d	37	c	38	c	39	d	40	a	41	c	42	b
43	c	44	b	45	b	46	b	47	a	48	b	49	c
50	d	51	d	52	d	53	b	54	a	55	c	56	a
57	c	58	b	59	b	60	d	61	d	62	c	63	c
64	d	65	c	66	b	67	c	68	d	69	a	70	a
71	c	72	b	73	a	74	c	75	b				

4

Gametogenesis

Rakesh Kumar Barhaiya

College of Veterinary Science & Animal Husbandry, Nanaji Deshmukh Veterinary Sciences University, Jabalpur, Madhya Pradesh

Introduction

Gametogenesis is the process by which gametes are produced in sexually reproducing organisms. This process involves a series of cellular divisions and differentiations and can be divided into two main types: spermatogenesis (the production of sperm) and oogenesis (the production of ova). Gametogenesis ensures genetic diversity through the processes of crossing over and independent assortment during meiosis. A gamete is a specialized cell involved in sexual reproduction. Gametes are haploid cells; contain only half the number of chromosomes of a diploid cell. Two gametes one from each parent fuses during fertilization to form a zygote, a diploid cell with a full set of chromosomes. The primordial germ cells develop from the wall yolk sac and differentiate into female and male gametes. During and after migration of primordial germ cells, they proliferate by mitoses and male and female primordial germ cells surrounded by somatic cells of their specific gonads and differentiate into oogonia in ovary and spermatogonia in testis. Meiosis is the process of cell division (Meiosis I and Meiosis II) in two specialized germ cells i.e. oogonia and spermatogonia to produce haploid female gametes (ovum) and male gametes (sperm) respectively. Meiosis I allow genetic recombination where exchange of DNA segment occurs between maternal and paternal chromatids.

Spermatogenesis

The development of sperm in the germinal epithelium of seminiferous tubules of the testis is known as spermatogenesis. Spermatogenesis starts, when the male animal attains the puberty. The sequential stages in spermatogenesis are

1. **Mitotic/multiplication phase:** Primordial germ cells undergo a series of mitotic divisions and localized in solid cords of primitive sustentacular cells (progenitor of Sertoli cells) within the seminiferous tubules (testis). At the age of puberty, the cell cords differentiated into seminiferous tubules of the testis and simultaneously primitive sustentacular cells became Sertoli cells and primordial germ cells produce spermatogonia throughout the life, having the features of stem cells. These spermatogonia remains dormant until the onset of puberty. Sertoli cells are very important for both physical support and paracrine regulation of spermatogenesis, and also form the blood-testis barrier by sealing off the seminiferous tubules with tight junctions. At puberty, they are activated and undergo series of mitotic division and produce clones of cells referred to as type A spermatogonia. Among type a

spermatogonia some cells divide and give rise to type B spermatogonia, from which primary spermatocytes are formed. Remaining type A spermatogonia cells will be retained for further spermatogenic cycle.

2. **Growth phase:** during this phase type B spermatogonia takes limited growth
3. **Maturation phase:** Type B spermatogonia produce diploid primary spermatocytes through mitotic division. The diploid primary spermatocytes undergo the Meiotic division I and form two haploid secondary spermatocyte. unlike oogenesis, it doesn't arrest at stage of dictyotene of prophase I. Each secondary spermatocyte divides into two spermatids through Meiotic division II. Thus, from one primary spermatocyte four spermatids are produced. So, from one type A spermatogonia, 16 primary spermatocytes and from which 64 spermatids are produced in each spermatogenic cycle.

Different phases of Spermatogenic cells from type A spermatogonia to spermatid is in close association with the Sertoli cells that means cytokinesis is incomplete and get nourishment and support from Sertoli cells. Sertoli cells helps in formation of blood-testis barrier through tight junction between adjacent Sertoli cells.

Spermiogenesis

A spermatid undergoes metamorphosis into a spermatozoon, that process is called spermiogenesis. A spermatid has all cell organelles of a typical mammalian cells like nucleus, Golgi apparatus, mitochondria, paired centrioles. This complex process is traditionally divided into four phases: the Golgi phase, the cap phase, the formation of the tail, and the maturation phase. During these stages, the cell undergoes significant morphological changes, including the development of the acrosome, flagellum, and the condensation of DNA within the nucleus. The result is a mature sperm cell, capable of fertilization after undergoing further maturation in the epididymis.

Golgi phase: The Golgi complex form multiple acrosomal granules, fused to form a single large acrosomal granule that becomes localized adjacent to the nucleus and the centrioles begin developing the tail.

Cap phase: The acrosomal granule flattens and reconstruct into the acrosome covers a larger portion of the anterior aspect of condensed nucleus and having hydrolysing enzymes that play important role in penetration of ovum during fertilization.

Tail phase: The centrioles migrated into the pole of the nucleus opposite the acrosome that form the axial filament from which the tail of the spermatozoon develops providing motility to the sperm cell. Mitochondria aggregate in the proximal region of the filament forming the middle piece of the spermatozoon.

Maturation phase: this is last phase spermiogenesis, where excess cytoplasm is shed (residual body), phagocytosed by Sertoli cell and species-specific shape (head and tail) is developed. Finally, spermatozoa ready for release from the Sertoli cells into the seminiferous tubules.

Spermiation: After spermiogenesis, immature spermatozoa are released from their intimate association with the Sertoli cells into the lumen of the seminiferous tubule that a process is called as spermiation. The spermatozoa within the seminiferous tubules are non-motile and are carried passively by the tubular fluid to the rete testis.

Maturation of spermatozoa: During their passage through epididymis spermatozoa undergo several changes; that enable them to become motile and capable of fertilization.

Structural Modifications: Spermatozoa develop disulfide bonds within their nucleus and tail, which enhance the structural integrity of the sperm membrane.

Surface Modifications: The sperm membrane undergoes significant changes, including the oxidation of sulfhydryl groups, which is essential for the stability and functionality of the sperm.

Acquisition of Motility: Initially immotile but when they leave the testes, spermatozoa gain progressive motility as they transit through the epididymis. This is facilitated by the unique environment created by the epididymal epithelium.

Fertilizing Ability: Spermatozoa acquire the ability to fertilize an egg during their passage through the epididymis. This involves changes in the sperm's surface proteins and the ability to undergo the acrosome reaction, which is crucial for penetrating the egg.

Environmental Adaptation: The epididymal fluid environment changes progressively along the length of the epididymis, providing the necessary conditions for sperm maturation. This includes the absorption and secretion of various proteins, enzymes, hormones, and other molecules.

These changes are essential for the sperm to become fully functional and capable of successful fertilization.

Oogenesis

Oogenesis is the process of producing and developing an ovum (egg cell) from primordial germ cells in the female reproductive system. Oogonia are the cells that arise from primordial germ cells in the ovary of foetus. They are formed through mitosis and are present in large numbers during early foetal development. The entire

ovary is covered by a germinal epithelium and from this the germinal cells dip into the cortex and multiply as oogonia which are surrounded by epithelial cells to produce follicles. Oogonia enlarges and enter the Prophase of 1st meiotic division and termed as primary oocytes (diploid) before birth. Primary oocytes surrounded by simple squamous epithelium of follicular cells, this structure called primordial follicle and remain in dictyotene stage of 1st meiotic division. During both the proliferative and resting phases, a high proportion of primordial follicles undergo atresia. At puberty, the oocyte increases in size and epithelial follicular cells form a stratified layer around the oocyte, known as a secondary follicle. Secondary follicle is surrounded by stratified epithelium of follicular cells (granulosa cells). Acellular layer of Glycoproteins (zona pellucida) secreted by inner granulosa cells between vitelline membrane and follicular cells. Stromal cells are proliferated and form multilayered spindle shaped theca cells around the granulosa cells. Tertiary follicle having primary oocytes remain attached by follicular wall by mass of granulosa cells called cumulus oophorus and fluid filled cavity (antrum) is formed. Oocytes surrounded by radially arranged columnar shape granulosa cell called corona radiata. Secondary oocytes (haploid) and first polar body is formed after completion of 1st meiotic division of primary oocytes just before ovulation. The secondary oocytes remain in suspended in metaphase stage of 2nd meiotic division until ovulation. Theca cells in tertiary follicle that surround the granulosa cell differentiated into an inner vascular theca interna and an outer layer of loose connective tissue of theca externa. After completion of 2nd meiotic division at the time of fertilization one ovum and second polar is formed.

Ovulation is the process where a mature egg is released from the ovary. The ovulation take place at ovulatory fossa of ovary in mare. Rupture follicle just after ovulation called corpus hemorrhagicum. Induced ovulation (by coitus) occurs in cat, rabbit, camel. Corpus luteum is formed and maintain if fertilization occurs. Regression of corpus luteum take place in the late diestrus and connective tissue scar is formed called corpus albicans.

Multiple Choice Questions

1. Gametogenesis occurs in which cells ....
   a) Hepatocytes b) Germ cells
   c) Somatic cell d) Leydig cells
2. Primordial germ cells develop from
   a) Yolk sac b) notochord
   c) mesentery d) All
3. Gametogenesis is the processes that includes
   a) Origin of primordial germ cells and their migration to the developing gonads
   b) Multiplication of germ cells in the gonad through the process of mitosis
   c) Reduction of the number of chromosomes by meiosis and maturation, differentiation of gametes into sperm in male and ova in female
   d) All
4. Spermatogenesis occurs in
   a) Germinal epithelium of seminiferous tubules
   b) Epithelium of epididymis
   c) Epithelium of vas efference
   d) None
5. The following statement is true for Spermatogenesis
   a) At, puberty, the dormant germ cells become activated and form spermatogonia type A through mitosis
   b) Spermatogonia type A form spermatogonia type B through mitosis from which primary spermatocytes arise
   c) Spermatogenesis occurs throughout the life
   d) All
6. Primary spermatocytes are..............
   a) Haploid cells
   b) Diploid cells
   c) Primary spermatocytes undergo meiosis I to form two secondary spermatocytes (haploid)
   d) Both and b and c
7. Primary spermatocytes are developed
   a) Prenatally b) At the time of birth
   c) Postnatally before puberty d) Postnatally after puberty

8. Secondary spermatocytes are
   a) Haploid cells which undergo meiosis II
   b) Each secondary spermatocytes produces two spermatids
   c) Both a and b
   d) None
9. Each spermatogenic cells produce ....spermatid (numbers)
   a) 8 b) 16
   c) 32 d) 64
10. The process of formation of spermatozoa from spermatid called......
   a) Metamorphosis of spermatid b) Spermiogenesis
   c) Activation d) Both a and b
11. The process of spermiogenesis includes
   a) Golgi complex form the proacrosomal granules and became fused to form acrosome
   b) The centrioles form axial filament opposite to the acrosome
   c) Mitochondria aggregate in the proximal region of the filament forming the middle piece of the spermatozoon.
   d) All
12. Spermiation is the process ....
   a) It is the process where spermatozoa released into the epididymis
   b) It is the process where spermatozoa released into vas deferens
   c) It is the process where spermatozoa released from Sertoli cells into lumen of seminiferous tubules
   d) None
13. The maturation process of spermatozoa occurs in ....
   a) Vas efference b) Vad deferens
   c) Epididymis d) All
14. Mature spermatozoa capable of fertilising oocytes are stored in .... prior to ejaculation
   a) Head of the epididymis b) Body of the epididymis
   c) Tail of epididymis d) None.
15. The process of oogenesis includes
   a) Proliferative phase where primordial germ cells produce oogonia
   b) Growth phase where oogonia enlarge and enter the Prophase of 1st meiotic division and termed as primary oocytes (diploid) before birth
   c) Maturation phase where secondary oocytes (haplod) formed after completion of 1st meiotic division of primary oocytes just before ovulation and formation of ovum after completion of 2nd meiotic division at the time of fertilization
   d) All

16. Primordial follicles are composed of.........
    a) Primary oocytes surrounded by simple squamous epithelium of follicular cells
    b) Primary oocytes remain in dictyotene stage of 1st meiotic division
    c) During both the proliferative and resting phases, a high proportion of primordial follicles undergo atresia)
    d) All
17. Secondary follicle are
    a) Multilaminar, having primary oocytes surrounded by stratified epithelium of follicular cells (granulosa cells)
    b) Acellular layer of Glycoproteins (zona pellucida) situated between vitelline membrane and follicular cells
    c) Secondary follicles don't have fluid filled cavity (antrum)
    d) All
18. Graafian or tertiary follicles are characterized by
    a) Fluid filled cavity (antrum) is formed
    b) Oocytes remain attached by follicular wall by mass of granulosa cells called cumulus oophorus
    c) In mature follicle, oocytes radially surrounded by columnar granulosa cells (corona radiata)
    d) All
19. One primary oocyte produces how many ova and polar bodies
    a) One ovum and two polar bodies b) One ovum and three polar bodies
    c) Two ovum and two polar bodies d) Two ovum and three polar bodies
20. Induced ovulation occurs in.......... species
    a) Rabbit b) Cat
    c) Camel d) all
21. In ....(species) 1st meiotic division is completed before ovulation
    a) cow b) mare
    c) bitch d) all
22. In ....(species) 1st meiotic division is completed after ovulation
    a) cow b) mare
    c) bitch d) botch b and c
23. The 2nd meiotic division of oocytes is arrested in
    a) Prophase b) Metaphase
    c) Anaphase d) Telophase
24. The division of arrested secondary oocytes (2nd meiotic division) is completed at
    a) Coitus b) Fertilization
    c) Ovulation d) None

265 After completion second meiotic division, one secondary oocyte gives

a) One ovum and one second polar body
b) One ovum and one first polar body
c) Two ovum and two second polar body
d) None

26. The ovum became ....when it fertilized

a) Zygote b) Morula
c) Blastula d) None

27. The degenerative process (regression) of ovarian follicles called

a) Depression b) Repletion
c) Atresia d) Deletion

28. Rupture follicle just after ovulation called

a) Corpus hemorrhagicum b) Corpus luteum
c) Corpus albicans d) None

29. Which cells are transformed into luteal cells during Luteinization

a) Granulosa cells b) Theca cells
c) Both a and b d) None

30. The connective tissue scar is present in regressed follicle is called

a) Corpus hemorrhagicum b) Corpus luteum
c) Corpus albicans d) None

31. Folliculogenesis is present in which part of ovary

a) Cortex b) Medulla
c) Both a and b d) None

32. Antrum is the characteristics features of the....................follicle

a) Primary follicle b) Secondary follicle
c) Tertiary follicle d) All

33. The oocytes of Graffian follicle lied on accumulation of granulosa cells that is called

a) Corona radiata b) Cumulous oophorus
c) Zona pellucida d) None

34. The primary oocytes remain in suspended in which stage of 1st meiotic division

a) Leptotene b) Zygotene
c) Pachytene d) Dictyotene

35. The secondary oocytes remain in suspended in which stage of 2nd meiotic division until ovulation....

a) Prophase b) Metaphase
c) Anaphase d) Telophase

36. The spermatozoa within the seminiferous tubules are
    a) Motile and actively move into the rete testis
    b) Motile and passively move into the rete testis by tubular fluid
    c) Immotile and passively move into the rete testis by tubular fluid
    d) None
37. Zona pellucida (Glycoprotein layer) is secreted by
    a) Cell membrane of oocytes
    b) Granulosa cells adjacent to the vitelline membrane
    c) Theca externa cells
    d) Theca interna cells
38. Which cells are the predecessors of the male and female gametes
    a) Primordial germ cells b) Somatic cells
    c) Oogonia d) All
39. Which type of cell division occurs during gametogenesis from primordial germ cells
    a) Mitosis b) Meiosis
    c) Amitosis d) Both a and b
40. Gametogenesis includes
    a) Recombination of genetic material
    b) Reduction of chromosome from diploid to haploid
    c) Cytodifferentiation
    d) All
41. Gametes have ………. number of chromosomes
    a) Haploid b) Diploid
    c) Triploid d) All
42. At the end of 1st meiotic division of oogenesis, the two daughter cells are formed and the larger daughter cells called
    a) Primary oocytes b) Secondary oocytes
    c) First polar body d) Second polar body
43. Unequal cell division during meiosis occurs in
    a) Oogenesis b) Spermatogenesis
    c) Both d) None
44. …………… the stage at which oocyte is generally ovulated in domestic animals except dog
    a) Prophase of meiosis I b) Metaphase of meiosis II
    c) Anaphase of meiosis II d) None
45. Hydrolytic enzymes are released from……………… (Part of spermatozoa) during fertilization
    a) Nucleus b) Midpiece
    c) Tail d) Acrosome

46. The head of the spermatozoa contains...
    a) Nucleus b) Acrosome
    c) Centriole d) Both a and b
47. The spermatogonia cells took their nourishment and support from
    a) Sertoli cells b) Leydig cells
    c) M cells d) Both a and b
48. The ovulation take place at..................of ovary in mare
    a) Ovulatory fossa b) Outer surface of ovary
    c) Hilus d) Both a and b
49. Testosterone hormones secreted by ......
    a) Sertoli cells b) Leydig cells
    c) M cells d) Luteal cell
50. Progesterone hormones secreted by ......
    a) Corpus luteum b) Corpus albicans
    c) Corpus hemorrhagicum d) All

Answer Key

1	b	2	a	3	d	4	a	5	d	6	d	7	d
8	c	9	d	10	d	11	d	12	c	13	c	14	c
15	d	16	d	17	d	18	d	19	d	20	a	21	a
22	d	23	b	24	b	25	a	26	a	27	c	28	a
29	c	30	c	31	a	32	c	33	b	34	d	35	b
36	c	37	b	38	a	39	d	40	d	41	a	42	b
43	a	44	b	45	d	46	d	47	a	48	a	49	b
50	a												

5

Fertilization

Jasvinder Singh Sasan[1], Shalini Suri[1], Kamal Sarma[1] and Anil Sharma[2]

[1]Division of Veterinary Anatomy, Faculty of Veterinary Sciences and Animal Husbandry, Sher-e-Kashmir University of Agricultural Sciences and Technology of Jammu, Jammu and Kashmir

[2]Department of Veterinary Anatomy, College of Veterinary Science & A.H., Kamdhenu University, Junagadh Campus, Gujarat

Introduction

Fertilization is sequence of events that begins with contact between a sperm and an oocyte, resulting in fusion of two gametes and formation of a zygote (unicellular embryo). ***Site of fertilization is distal end of ampulla of fallopian tube (ampulla-isthmus junction) in mammals and in birds, is infundibulum.*** Only 1% of sperms deposited in vagina enter cervix. Movement of sperm from cervix to uterine tube occurs by muscular contractions of uterus & uterine tube and by their own propulsion.

Immediately after ovulation, ovum is caught by the fimbriae of the infundibular part of oviduct and is brought to the ampulla.Cilia along epithelium of oviduct moves OCc.

In farm animals (except swine) corona radiata cells drop off in ampulla. In swine, they persist and help in attachment of ova to each other in forming egg-clumps. The optimum fertilizable life of egg in most mammals is 12-24 hours after ovulation, but in dog it may extend up to 4 days.

Site of ejaculation is

Cow, primates, sheep, goat: Anterior vagina

Horse, pig: Body of uterus

Capacitation

Spermatozoa are not able to fertilize the oocyte immediately after arrival in female genital tract. To acquire fertility, they must reside there for a certain period of time. The changes that occur during this period constitute **capacitation.** Ejaculated spermatozoa must be exposed to secretions of female reproductive tract for a variable period of time before they attain capacity to fertilize oocyte. The secretions of uterus & oviduct participate in capacitation. Important processes during capacitation are:

1. Surface of spermatozoa in region of epididymis acquires certain molecules (proteins & carbohydrates in nature) and in seminal plasma, these molecules are masked by surface proteins. In female reproductive tract, these molecules along with surface proteins are removed. Removal of cholesterol and GAGs sperm cell surface.

2. Destabilization of sperm plasma membrane which is phospholipid bilayer by cholesterol efflux. This destabilized PM of sperm increases calcium permeability.
3. Elevation of intracellular pH and bicarbonate levels to stimulate cAMP production which helps in hyperactivity of sperm.
4. Activation of receptor sites present on sperm head
5. Activation of acrosomal enzymes.

Sperm hyperactivity

At 1st, sperm moves in serpentine motion. Once in uterine cavity, sperm motility becomes hyperactivated and whip-like. This change allows sperm to negotiate through cumulus layer and zona pellucida)

Binding of zona pellucida

Receptors on sperm plasma membrane bind to ZP3 only which initiate acrosome reaction.

Acrosome reaction

Once sperm binds zona pellucida, it undergoes **acrosome reaction.** It is release of acrosomal contents. It involves fusion of outer acrosome membrane with sperm plasma membrane resulting in formation of vesicles through which acrosomal enzymes are released causing lysis of zona pellucida. Acrosome reaction is indicator of complete capacitation. Acrosin & hyaluronidase are enzymes released during acrosome reaction. Acrosin hydrolyze ZP proteins and enhances the ability of spermatozoa to binds these proteins.

Binding and penetration of oolemma

After penetrating ZP, sperm fuses with the plasma membrane (oolemma) of the oocyte. Membrane oocyte fuses with equatorial segment of spermatozoa. Oolemma contains microvilli on its surface. Equatorial region on sperm head fuses with microvilli on oolemma. Once equatorial region on sperm head is fused with plasma membrane of oocyte, microvilli engulf sperm. Sperm head and tail enters the oocyte cytoplasm, but its plasma membrane is left behind. With entry of sperm nucleus in oocyte cytoplasm, meiosis-II is resumed resulting in release of polar bodies and oocyte.

Immediately after the entry of spermatozoa, oocyte undergoes **oocyte activation.** After adhesion, fusion of plasma membrane takes place. Fusion is between plasma membrane of oocyte and membrane that covers posterior region of sperm head. Both head and tail of sperm enters cytoplasm of oocyte but not plasma membrane. Egg responds in 3 ways:

1. Release of 2nd polar body

Prior to fertilization, egg is in quiescent state, arrested in metaphase of M-II. Upon binding of sperm, M-II resumes with release of 2nd polar body.

2. Cortical reaction

Immediately after fertilization, ovum surface changes to prevent fusion of additional spermatozoa. When this mechanism fails, polyspermic fertilization can result with formation of polyploidy embryos that undergo embryonic death. Polyspermy is common in birds and reptiles. Block is provided by cortical reaction.

When spermatozoa enter peri-vitelline space, cortical granules migrate to periphery of oocyte and release content by exocytosis. These granules are present beneath plasma membrane. Sperm entry initiates fusion of cortical granule membrane with egg cell membrane. Cortical granule contents are:

1. Serine protease: It dissolve protein connections between envelop and membrane. It clips off receptors and connected sperm
2. Mucopolysaccharides
3. Peroxidases: Hardens fertilization envelop
4. Hyaline proteins: Form coating around egg called hyaline layer

Cortical granule causes

a) Extensive reorganization of zona pellucida ZP becomes impermeable and prevents entry of excess spermatozoa in peri-vitelline space. This is called **zona reaction.**

b) Causes thickening of peri-vitelline space so that fusion of excess sperm and oolemma are prevented. This is called **vitelline block.**

3. Metabolic activation of egg

Formation of male pronucleus. Tail detaches and disintegrates. Male and female pronuclei fuses, loose nuclear envelope and forms zygote. Mixing of male and female pronuclei is called **karyogamy or synkaryosis.** It enters 1st mitotic division. 1st cleavage is normally seen within 24 hours after ovulation. Pronucleus is name used for nucleus of sperm & egg, after sperm enters ovum but before they fuses.

Multiple Choice Questions

1. Site of fertilization in birds:
   a) Magnum b) Infundibulum
   c) Isthmus d) Ampulla
2. Site of ejaculation in ruminants is:
   a) Body of uterus b) Posterior vagina
   c) Anterior vagina d) Uterine horns
3. Site of ejaculation in equines is:
   a) Body of uterus b) Posterior vagina
   c) Anterior vagina d) Uterine horns
4. Site of ejaculation in pig is:
   a) Body of uterus b) Posterior vagina
   c) Anterior vagina d) Uterine horns
5. In which of the following species, volume of ejaculate is large and is divided into pre-sperm, sperm rich and post-sperm fraction:
   a) Cattle b) Goat
   c) Pig d) All of the above
6. Uterus is the site of deposition of spermatozoa in all except:
   a) Dog b) Horse
   c) Cattle d) All of the above
7. Vagina is the site of deposition of spermatozoa in all except:
   a) Horse b) Cattle
   c) Sheep d) Humans

8. Proportion of male to female zygotes which result from fertilization in mammals is known as:
   a) Primary sex ratio b) Secondary sex ratio
   c) Tertiary sex ratio d) None of the above
9. The proportion of male to female animals at birth is known as:
   a) Primary sex ratio b) Secondary sex ratio
   c) Tertiary sex ratio d) None of the above
10. Avian spermatozoa contain:
   a) W chromosome only b) Z chromosome only
   c) Either Z or W chromosome d) None of the above
11. Sperm lysin, the enzymatic substance produced by sperms in mammals is known as:
   a) Cryanogamone b) Hyaluronic acid
   c) Androgamone d) Hyaluronidase
12. Egg development without fertilization is known as:
   a) Parthenogenesis b) Metagenesis
   c) Oogenesis d) Gametogenesis
13. After a sperm has penetrated an ovum in the process of fertilization, entry of further sperms is prevented by:
   a) Condensation of yolk b) Zona reaction
   c) Vitelline block d) Both b and c
14. Which of the following is true regarding the process of fertilization:
   a) Entry of sperm activates the egg for completing meiosis
   b) Only one sperm reaches the egg and enters it
   c) Only the acrosome of the sperm enters the egg
   d) All of the above
15. Minute cell which separates from the animal egg during maturation is known as:
   a) Primary oogonia b) Secondary oogonia
   c) Polar body d) Primary spermatogonia
16. Which of the following helps sperm in penetrating egg:
   a) Antifertilizin b) Sperm lysin
   c) Fertilizin d) None of the above
17. In mammals, fertilization occurs in:
   a) Penis b) Oviduct
   c) Ovary d) Vasa deferentia
18. External fertilization occurs in:
   a) Humans b) Amphibians
   c) Mammals d) Dogs
19. Zona pellucida is composed of ____________ glycoproteins:
   a) ZP10 b) ZP11
   c) ZP3 d) ZP5

20. What occurs when egg and sperm fuse?
    a) Differentiation b) Development
    c) Fertilization d) Cleavage
21. In animal cell, which organelle is only provided by sperm to the oocyte following fertilization:
    a) Peroxisomes b) Mitochondria
    c) Centrioles d) All of the above
22. In most of the animal species, the mitochondria of zygote is predominantly derived from:
    a) Oocyte b) Sperm
    c) Both a & b d) None of the above
23. In mammals, which protein is crucial for the recognition and binding of sperm to the egg, facilitating fertilization:
    a) Bindin b) Resact
    c) Izumo d) Ovastacin
24. Sperm ____________, which helps in penetrating egg during fertilization in mammals, contains ________________:
    a) Lysin, hyaluronidase b) Fertilizin, hyaluronidase
    c) Lysin, hyaluronic acid d) Fertilizin, hyaluronic acid
25. What is karyogamy:
    a) Fusion of gametic nucleus b) Fusion of gametoplasm
    c) Fusion of gametes d) None of the above
26. Which of the following is not a function of fertilizin-antifertilizin reaction:
    a) Sperm identifies egg
    b) Release hyaluronidase
    c) Fertilization between different species is prevented
    d) None of the above
27. Which part of sperm helps in its entry into the cytoplasm of the ovum:
    a) Plasma membrane b) Neck
    c) Nucleus d) Acrosome
28. Fertilized egg is known as:
    a) Germ cell b) Embryo
    c) Zygote d) Blastula
29. Which of the following process related to sperm occurs in female reproductive tract:
    a) Maturation b) Spermiation
    c) Capacitation d) Spermatocytogeneis
30. Maturation of sperm takes place when sperm travels through:
    a) Epididymis b) Oviduct
    c) Cervix d) Urethra

31. Which of the following changes are associated with capacitation of sperm:
   a) Efflux of sterols b) Increase level of cAMP
   c) Ca^{2+} influx d) All of the above
32. The correct sequence of events in fertilization is:
   a) Capacitation, zona binding, acrosome reaction, cortical reaction
   b) Capacitation, acrosome reaction, zona binding, cortical reaction
   c) Capacitation, zona binding, cortical reaction, acrosome reaction
   d) Acrosome reaction, zona binding, capacitation, cortical reaction
33. Contents of cortical granules is/are:
   a) Peroxidases b) Hyaline proteins
   c) Serine protease d) All of the above
34. Freshly ejaculated mammalian sperm are unable to fertilize eggs in vivo until they had resided for a period of time within the female reproductive tract. This was observed by:
   a) Karl von Baer b) Chang and Austin
   c) Haeckel d) Leeuwenhoek
35. Which hormone promotes muscular activity of the female tubular genitalia to assist with spermatozoa transport:
   a) ADH b) Oxytocin
   c) Relaxin d) Somatostatin
36. Which specific protein in the zona serves as a binding site for spermatozoa:
   a) ZP1 b) ZP2
   c) ZP3 d) ZP10
37. Which cell organelle is associated with formation of acrosome:
   a) Mitochondria b) Golgi complex
   c) Endoplasmic reticulum d) Centrioles
38. Capacitation of the sperm:
   a) Caused by zona pellucida b) Occurs in male
   c) Prevents polyspermy d) Essential for fertilization
39. Among following, which is pre-fertilization event:
   a) Zygote formation b) Gametogenesis
   c) Syngamy d) Embryogenesis
40. External fertilization is seen in all of these except:
   a) Mammals b) Fishes
   c) Amphibians d) All of the above
41. What role does the acrosome have in fertilization:
   a) It responds to egg's chemoattractants
   b) It has enzymes that digest the zona pellucida
   c) It has enzymes that digest the nuclear membrane
   d) It is the part of the egg that prevents sperm from binding

42. ZZ/ZW designation of chromosomes is used in:
 a) Avian b) Fish
 c) Reptiles d) All of the above
43. The interval between fertilization and implantation in mare is about:
 a) 4 to 5 days b) 5 to 10 days
 c) 10 to 20 days d) 20 to 50 days
44. The fertilization in mammals occurs in:
 a) Ampulla of oviduct b) Infundibulum of oviduct
 c) Isthmus of oviduct d) Uterine horn
45. The factor affects the retrograde loss of spermatozoa from the female genital tract is:
 a) Physical nature of ejaculate
 b) Volume of ejaculate
 c) Site of deposition in female genital tract
 d) All of these
46. The unfertilized ovum can remains for months in the oviduct of:
 a) Cow b) Bitch
 c) Mare d) Sow
47. What is androgenesis?
 a) Abnormal fertilization without genetic contribution from oocytes
 b) Abnormal fertilization in which only male pronucleus develops
 c) Both a & b
 d) Normal fertilization without genetic contribution from sperm
48. Which of the following statement is NOT true for capacitation of spermatozoa:
 a) Capacitation of spermatozoa is essential for fertilization
 b) Removal of glycoprotein coat and seminal plasma proteins from sperm surface
 c) Flagellar motility of sperm is altered
 d) Capacitation of all spermatozoa occurs at the same time
49. When more than one sperm participates in fertilization, the process is known as:
 a) Polygamy b) Polyspermy
 c) Parthenogenesis d) None of these
50. In mammals the polyspermy is leads to:
 a) Death of embryo
 b) Normal development of embryo
 c) Defective development of embryo
 d) Development of new species
51. The polyspermy is a normal phenomenon in fertilization process of:
 a) Pig b) Birds
 c) Horses d) Cattle

52. The zona reaction is ineffective to prevent the polyspermy in:
    a) Cattle b) Sheep
    c) Rabbit d) Dog
53. Following natural mating, the fertilization rate in dogs, cats and pigs ranges from:
    a) 70% to 80% b) 70% to 90%
    c) 80% to 90% d) 85% to 100%
54. The ovulated mammalian egg consists of:
    a) Only oocyte with zona pellucida
    b) Only oocyte without zona pellucida
    c) Oocyte with zona pellucida and cumulus cells
    d) Oocyte without zona pellucida and with cumulus cells
55. The transportation of spermatozoa in female reproductive tract, occurs in:
    a) One phase b) Two phases
    c) Three phases d) None of these

Answer Key

1	b	2	c	3	a	4	a	5	c	6	c	7	a
8	a	9	b	10	b	11	d	12	a	13	d	14	a
15	c	16	b	17	b	18	b	19	c	20	c	21	c
22	a	23	c	24	a	25	a	26	b	27	d	28	c
29	c	30	a	31	d	32	a	33	d	34	b	35	b
36	c	37	b	38	d	39	b	40	a	41	b	42	d
43	d	44	a	45	d	46	c	47	c	48	d	49	b
50	a	51	b	52	c	53	d	54	c	55	b		

6

Cleavage and Blastulation

Jasvinder Singh Sasan, Kamal Sarma and Shalini Suri

Division of Veterinary Anatomy, Faculty of Veterinary Sciences and Animal Husbandry, Sher-e-Kashmir University of Agricultural Sciences and Technology of Jammu, Jammu and Kashmir

Introduction

Cleavage is the process of cellular division without growth. It is also called segmentation division and it follows immediately after fertilization. By the end of this process, single cell zygote is transformed into multi-cellular stage called blastula. Daughter cells are called blastomeres. All divisions are mitotic and occur consequently. Ratio of nucleus to cytoplasm is very low at beginning but later they resemble somatic cell. Cleavage division always start at animal pole. Cleavage can be classified as:

1. **Holoblastic/Total cleavage:** Whole fertilized ovum is involved in production of blastomere. It is also called complete cleavage.
    a) **Equal:** All blastomeres are of equal size. E.g. mammals
    b) **Unequal:** Some blastomeres at vegetal pole are larger. E.g. amphibians
2. **Meroblastic/Partial cleavage:** When deutoplasm is abundant and only a part of fertilized ovum is involved in cleavage, it is called meroblastic cleavage.
    a) **Discoidal:** Cleavage is confined to the germinal disc i.e. at animal pole. E.g. birds and reptiles.
    b) **Superficial:** Cleavage is confined to the peripheral margin of cytoplasm. E.g. arthropods.

Dividing continuously, embryo attains a stage of 16-32 cells. 16-celled stage is called early/uncompact morula and 32-celled stage is called compact morula. This stage is called morula due to its close resemblance to mulberry fruit. Structure is surrounded by zona pellucida.

After morula stage, fluid accumulation begins and blastomeres are gradually pushed to the periphery. As fluid accumulation progresses further, it leads to formation of large cavity in central part of embryo known as ***blastocoels*** and morula stage is now transformed into ***blastula/blastocyst stage.*** Blastomeres now arrange themselves as single celled outer layer called ***trophoblast*** and small group of cells at animal pole called ***inner cell mass (ICM).*** Trophoblasts give rise to fetal membranes and will help embryo in its attachment to uterine wall (implantation). ICM gives rise to all organs of body. Development of blastula is called ***blastulation.***

Multiple Choice Questions

1. The blastocoele becomes:
   a) Amniotic cavity b) Extra-embryonic coelom
   c) Primary Yolk sac d) Secondary cavity
2. Meroblastic cleavage is a division which is:
   a) Horizontal b) Partial
   c) Total d) Spiral
3. Type of cleavage seen in birds:
   a) Holoblastic and equal b) Meroblastic and discoidal
   c) Holoblastic and discoidal d) Meroblastic and superficial
4. Type of cleavage seen in mammals:
   a) Equal holoblastic b) Unequal holoblastic
   c) Discoidal meroblastic d) Superficial meroblastic
5. Type of cleavage seen in amphibians:
   a) Equal holoblastic b) Unequal holoblastic
   c) Discoidal meroblastic d) Superficial meroblastic
6. Type of cleavage seen in arthropods:
   a) Equal holoblastic b) Unequal holoblastic
   c) Discoidal meroblastic d) Superficial meroblastic
7. The ratio of cells in Inner cell mass to those in the trophoectoderm is:
   a) 1:1 b) 1:2
   c) 1:3 d) 1:4
8. In which species, a compensatory capsule is formed between trophoectoderm and the overlying zona pellucida before zona is shed:
   a) Mare b) Cow
   c) Bitch d) Pig
9. In birds, embryo develops from:
   a) Area pellucida b) Area opaqa
   c) Area vasculosa d) Koller's sickle
10. The portion of the trophoectoderm covering the Inner cell mass is known as:
    a) Mural trophoblast b) Polar trophoblast
    c) Hypoblast d) Somite
11. Around the time of zona hatching, which of the following differentiates into epiblast & hypoblast:
    a) Polar trophoblast b) Mural trophoblast
    c) Inner cell mass d) Zona pellucida
12. In mammals, the type of egg is:
    a) Alecithal b) Microlecithal
    c) Mesolecithal d) Macrolecithal

13. Central translucent area in blastodisc in chick is called:
    a) Area pellucida b) Area opaqa
    c) Area vasculosa d) Koller's sickle
14. Peripheral darker area in blastodisc in chick is called:
    a) Area pellucida b) Area opaqa
    c) Area vasculosa d) Koller's sickle
15. Which of the following area is not seen in the blastodisc of chick:
    a) Area pellucida b) Area magna
    c) Area vasculosa d) Area opaqa
16. Plane of cleavage which passes through median axis of egg from animal to vegetal pole is:
    a) Meridional plane b) Vertical plane
    c) Equatorial plane d) Horizontal plane
17. Plane of cleavage which passes from the animal pole to the vegetal pole, but does not pass through the median axis of the egg is:
    a) Meridional plane b) Vertical plane
    c) Equatorial plane d) Horizontal plane
18. Plane of cleavage which bisects the egg at right angles to the median axis half way between the animal and vegetal poles is:
    a) Meridional plane b) Vertical plane
    c) Equatorial plane d) Horizontal plane
19. The fluid-filled cavity in blastula is known as:
    a) Blastopore b) Blastocoel
    c) Blastomere d) Blastodisc
20. Which of the following is not a characteristic feature of cleavage:
    a) All divisions are mitotic
    b) Process ends with formation of blastocoels
    c) Cleavage division always start at animal pole
    d) Cleavage division always start at vegetal pole
21. Type of blastula seen in birds is:
    a) Discoblastula b) Periblastula
    c) Stereoblastula d) Coeloblastula
22. Type of blastula seen in arthropods is:
    a) Discoblastula b) Periblastula
    c) Stereoblastula d) Coeloblastula
23. Type of blastula seen in amphibians is:
    a) Discoblastula b) Periblastula
    c) Stereoblastula d) Coeloblastula

24. Stage of cleavage where the blastomeres are completely arranged inside the zona pellucida giving a mulberry fruit shape is known as:
    a) Blastomere b) Blastula
    c) Morula d) Primitive yolk sac
25. Stage of embryo used for embryo transfer in ETT (Embryo Transfer Technology) is:
    a) 16 celled stage b) 8 celled stage
    c) 32 celled stage d) 64 celled stage
26. In sheep, totipotency of blastomeres is maintained up to:
    a) 16 celled stage b) 8 celled stage
    c) 32 celled stage d) 64 celled stage
27. In which species, only embryos are allowed to enter the uterus while unfertilized oocytes are retained in the oviduct:
    a) Mare b) Cattle
    c) Bitch d) Pig
28. In the domestic species, which of the following form Rauber's layer:
    a) Mural trophoblast b) Polar trophoblast
    c) Hypoblast d) Epiblast
29. Which law state that "The speed or rate of cleavage in any region of egg is inversely proportional to the amount of yolk it contains":
    a) Sach's law b) Baer's law
    c) Germ plasm theory d) Balfour's law
30. Which law state that "Each new division plane tends to intersect the preceding plane at right angles":
    a) Sach's law b) Baer's law
    c) Germ plasm theory d) Balfour's law
31. The simplest pattern of cleavage, in which successful division planes are at 90 degree angles relative to each other is:
    a) Spiral cleavage b) Radial cleavage
    c) Holoblastic cleavage d) Meroblastic cleavage
32. Cleavage which is characteristic of Deutrostomes and results in indeterminant cells is:
    a) Spiral cleavage b) Radial cleavage
    c) Both a & b d) None of the above
33. Cleavage which is characteristic of Protostomes and results in determinant cells is:
    a) Spiral cleavage b) Radial cleavage
    c) Both a & b d) None of the above
34. Which of the following is incorrect regarding radial cleavage:
    a) Successful division planes are at 90 degree angles relative to each other
    b) Characteristic of Deutrostomes
    c) Characteristic of Protostomes
    d) Results in indeterminant cells

35. Which of the following is incorrect regarding spiral cleavage:
 a) Characteristic of Deutrostomes b) Characteristic of Protostomes
 c) Results in determinant cells d) Both b & c
36. Determinate cleavage is seen in all except:
 a) Annelids b) Mollusks
 c) Ascidians d) Echinoderms
37. Indeterminate cleavage is seen in:
 a) Annelids b) Mollusks
 c) Ascidians d) Echinoderms
38. During cleavage in bird egg, subgerminal space is formed between:
 a) Blastoderm and yolk b) Epiblast and hypoblast
 c) Hypoblast and yolk d) None of the above
39. During cleavage in bird egg, blastocoel is formed between:
 a) Blastoderm and yolk b) Epiblast and hypoblast
 c) Hypoblast and yolk d) None of the above
40. Which of the following is also known as meroblastic cleavage:
 a) Superficial b) Equal
 c) Discoidal d) Partial
41. Discoidal and superficial are which types of cleavage:
 a) Equal holoblastic b) Unequal holoblastic
 c) Both a & b d) Meroblastic
42. How many cleavages are completed in the 16-celled stage of an egg?
 a) 12 b) 4
 c) 8 d) 3
43. The spindle in the determinate cleavage is:
 a) Horizontal b) Oblique
 c) Vertical d) Equatorial
44. The fertilized egg divides by the process of:
 a) Regeneration b) Gastrulation
 c) Invagination d) Cleavage
45. In the process of cleavage, the egg:
 a) Does not divide but only increase in size
 b) Divides repeatedly but without growth
 c) Divides repeatedly and grows
 d) None of the above
46. Cleavage differs from normal mitotic division in:
 a) There is no nuclear division during cleavage
 b) There is no division of the cytoplasm during cleavage
 c) There is no period of growth in between the divisions
 d) The division of the cytoplasm follows nuclear divisions

47. Blastula which is solid is:
 a) Discoblastula b) Superficial blastula
 c) Stereoblastula d) Coeloblastula
48. The eggs in which fate of every part of the egg becomes fixed are called:
 a) Cleidoic eggs b) Non-cleidoic eggs
 c) Regulative eggs d) Mosaic eggs
49. In spiral cleavage turn of spiral may be:
 a) Clockwise b) Anti-clockwise
 c) Both a & b d) None of the above
50. The ratio of the nucleus to cytoplasm at the beginning of cleavage is:
 a) Very high b) Normal
 c) Very low d) Higher than normal

Answer Key

1	c	2	b	3	b	4	a	5	b	6	d	7	c
8	a	9	a	10	b	11	c	12	a	13	a	14	b
15	b	16	a	17	b	18	c	19	b	20	d	21	a
22	b	23	d	24	c	25	c	26	b	27	a	28	b
29	d	30	a	31	b	32	b	33	a	34	c	35	a
36	d	37	d	38	a	39	b	40	d	41	d	42	b
43	b	44	d	45	b	46	c	47	c	48	d	49	c
50	c												

7

Gastrulation

Varsha Gupta and M.M. Farooqui

Department of Veterinary Anatomy, College of Veterinary Science and Animal Husbandry, U. P. Pt. Deen Dayal Upadhyaya Pashu Chikitsa Vigyan Vishwavidyalaya Evam Go-Anusandhan Sansthan (DUVASU), Mathura-281001, Uttar Pradesh

Introduction

Gastrulation is a vital stage in the development of multicellular animals because it establishes the basic body plan, including the primary body axes (dorsal/ventral axis and the cranial/caudal axis) and prepares the embryo for organ formation. The process of cleavage leads to formation of blastula which is followed by gastrulation. The blastula consists of inner cell mass (Cell mass made up of darker blastomere and present at animal pole which is going to form embryo proper) and trophoblast (Cells made up of clear cells and arranged periphery near to Zona pellucid). The morphogenic changes occur during gastrulation is the formation of three germ layers. Gastrulation is the process in which single- layered blastula is converted into a trilaminar structure consisting of an outer ectodermal, a middle mesodermal and an inner endodermal layer and occupy their characteristic position in embryo. They will be give rise to different organs and extra embryonic membranes. The gastrulation is an important step of cell differentiation.

Gastrulation in Mammals

The process of gastrulation is variable among different domestic animals. It takes place in the uterus when the blastocyst is floating in the uterine fluid. After the degeneration of zona – pellucida, the cells located in the ventral margin of the inner cell mass separate out and extended ventrally along the trophoblast layer. Due to further proliferation, splitting (delaminate) and migration of cells from the inner cell mass, form a complete cellular lining on the inner site of trophoblast. This newly formed layer is called endoderm corresponds to the hypoblast of chick blastoderm. The remaining cells of the inner cell mass correspond to the epiblast of chick blastoderm. With formation of endoderm the blastocoel is divided into 2 cavities. The portion enclosed within endoderm is called primitive gut and area between endoderm and trophoblast layer is extra embryonic coelom. During this time trophoblast cells covering the inner cell mass degenerate and compact inner cell mass exposed and it is called as embryonic disc The embryonic disc occupies a position at the animal pole.

Note: The development of the germ layers in mammals closely resembles that of birds with the formation of the primitive streak and primitive node.

After formation of endoderm blastocyst undergoes elongation. The cells of embryonic disc on the epiblast surface (surface cell layer) rapidly proliferates cephalo - caudal axis of developing embryo. This midline thicken area of embryonic disc is called primitive streak. When, primitive streak is fully developed than two marginal elevations called Primitive ridge and central groove called as primitive groove are developed)

At the cephalic end of primitive groove a cluster of tightly packed cell is present called Henson'snode or Primitive knot. The primitive streak is an area of rapid cellular growth and multiplication. The majority of migrating cells enter the coelom as primary mesenchyme. The newly formed cells spread ventro – laterally between endoderm and embryonic disc and become mesoderm.

In primitive streak, size of superficial cell layer is larger than other cells types. The superficial cell layer forms the ectoderm layer, which are continuous with trophoblast cells layer. These trophoblast cells layer are called as tropho-ectoderm.

Formation of Notochord

The cells of Hensen's node proliferate and migrate ventrally and formed cylindrical rod like structure in central midline, anterior to primitive streak in the area free of mesodermal cell. This rod shaped mass of cell is called notochord (Notochord is a rod like rostral extension of primitive node which extends from the cranial to caudal region ventral to the developing neural tube). It defines the cranial – caudal axis of embryo proper. It serves as inductor/ precursor for the formation of head process, nervous system and formation of somites. The base of the cranium and future location of the vertebral column are mark by the notochord. Cells which are present near the midline of the ectodermal layer elongate to form the neural plate, induced by the proximity of the notochord, a rod of mesodermal cells. The neural plate folds inwards and seals to form the neural tube. Some neuro- ectodermal cells migrate from the lateral margin of the developing neural tube and occupy dorso-lateral position to neural tube. These cells are called as neural crest cells. Neural tube gives rise to CNS. The PNS develops from both the neural tube and neural crest cells.

The mesodermal cell layer expands laterally beyond the limit of embryonic disc along with tropho- ectoderm. The developing mesoderm is arranged into three distinct areas.

a) Paraxial mesoderm: Mesoderm adjacent to the developing neural tube forms a thickened column of cells referred to as paraxial mesoderm. The cells of dorsal or paraxial mesoderm between cephalic and caudal ends of embryo arranged into block like masses, somites. Somites are mesodermal segmented blocks situated on either side of neural tube. The first pair of somite appears at 20 days post fertilization in cow, 17 days post fertilization in sheep, 13 days post fertilization in pig and 22 hours of incubation in chicks. Somites first appear in head region and are added progressively towards tail. Initially somites are solid masses of cells. During development of embryo a small cavity is formed in center of somite called as myocoele. Latter somites, distinctively arranged into three separate masses of cell which are-

    1) Sclerotome: The cells of ventral part of somite mixed with cells of myocoele and form sclerotome, which give rise to vertebrae, ribs, basilar part of sphenoid and occipital bones.

    2) Dermotome–The cells of dorso lateral part of somite form dermatome which give rise to axial muscle and skin.

3) Myotome: The remaining cells of somite at its dorso medial part are called myotome, which give rise to muscles of axial and appendicular skeleton.

b) Intermediate cell mass/ Nephrotome–: Mesoderm lateral to the somites forms a column of cells referred to as intermediate mesoderm. It is present in between the paraxial mesoderm and lateral plate mesoderm. It gives rise to uro- genital system.

c) Lateral plate mesoderm: In lateral plate mesoderm small cavities are present. All the small cavities combine to form a large cavity called as intraembryonic coelom. This intraembryonic coelom forms the pericardial sac, pleural sac and peritoneal sac. After the development of intra-embryonic coelom the lateral plate mesoderm divides into a parietal layer called as somatic mesoderm (forms lateral and ventral body walls of the embryo except musculature and ribs) and the visceral layer called as splanchnic mesoderm (forms most of the Gatro intestinal tract located in thorax and abdomen and lungs).

The membrane made up of ectoderm and somatic mesoderm is the somatopleure and that made up of endoderm and splanchnic mesoderm is the splanchanopleure. The space between the layers is the coelom. Somatopleurae forms lateral and ventral body walls of embryo except musculature and ribs that are derived from migrating somite cells and continues beyond embryos as amnion and chorion. Splanehnopleurae forms most of the G1 tract located in thorax and abdomen and lungs and is continuous with yolk sac in young embryos.

Derivatives of germ layers: The ectoderm gives rise to the nervous system and sense organs, the lining of the oral and nasal cavities, the epidermal structures of the skin and tip and body of the tongue. The endoderm forms the epithelial structures (lining and glands) of the respiratory and digestive systems, pharynx, root of tongue, Eustachian tube, tonsil, larynx, trachea, lungs, oesophagus, stomach, intestine liver, gall bladder, pancreas, urinary bladder, part of vagina, urethra, prostate and Cowper's gland. Most of the structures of the cardiovascular system, lymphoid tissue (spleen, lymphnode), body cavities and serous membranes, notochord, most of the connective tissue including cartilages, bones, joints and muscular tissue and urinary and genital system are derivatives of mesoderm.

Multiple Choice Questions

1. Which of the following is the process of formation of three germ layers?

   a) Cleavage b) Gastrulation

   c) Fertilization d) Implantation

2. The primordia of pancreas lie originally in the

   a) Ventral mesentery b) Dorsal mesentery

   c) Dorsal and ventral mesenteries d) Not included in mesentery

3. Most superficial foetal membrane is

   a) Yolk sac b) Amnion

   c) Chorion d) Allantois

4. Which of the following give rise to first angioblast?

   a) Yolk sac b) Chorion

   c) Fetal bone marrow d) Amnion

5. Myoepithelial cells are derived from
   a) Ectoderm of head b) Mesoderm
   c) Ectoderm of neural crest d) All of the above
6. Cerebral hemispheres develop from:
   a) Meten cephalon b) Telen cephalon
   c) Mylen cephalon d) Dien cephalon
7. Stapes develops from which of the branchial arch :
   a) I b) II
   c) III d) IV
8. Hair and sweat glands develop from :
   a) Mesoderm b) Ectoderm
   c) Endoderm d) None of the above
9. Blood tinged mucous discharge from uterus for about one month after parturition is called as
   a) Luchia b) Placenta
   c) First water bag d) All of the above
10. Rotation, herniation, coiling, reentry and placement are observed in the development of :
    a) Stomach b) Intestine
    c) Liver d) Pharynx
11. The condition of congenital absence of hair is known as:
    a) Agnathia b) Athelia
    c) Amelia d) Atrichia
12. When amount of amniotic fluid exceeds than normal, the condition is called:
    a) Oligohydromnion b) Aminotitis
    c) Polyhydramnions d) hydrogravide
13. In which process do the cells became progressively smaller
    a) Cleavage b) Morphogenesis
    c) Growth d) Differentiation
14. Epithelial lining of digestive and respiratory tract, urinary bladder and urethra are derived from
    a) Ectoderm b) Endoderm
    c) Mesoderm d) Chorionic villi
15. The part of sperm containing proteolytic enzymes to digest zona pellucida is
    a) Capacitor b) Cornea
    c) Head d) Acrosome
16. In which week of gestation (mammals) primitive streak appears first
    a) First b) Second
    c) Third d) fourth

17. Germ layer from which Cardiac development takes place is
    a) Ectoderm b) Somatic mesoderm
    c) Splanchnic mesoderm d) Endoderm
18. The outermost foetal membrane is
    a) Yolk sac b) Allantois
    c) Amnion d) Chorion
19. Sclerotome forms the ______________
    a) Vertebra b) Ribs
    c) Muscles d) Both a & b
20. Major part of the muscular system is formed by ______________
    a) Myotome b) Sclerotome
    c) Primitive gut d) Ectoderm
21. Development of the skeletal muscle involves the differentiation of myotome cells into________________
    a) Osteoblasts b) Myoblast
    c) Neural tube d) Neural crest
22. Skeletal muscles are derived from ___________
    a) Ectoderm b) Endoderm
    c) Mesoderm d) All of these
23. Skeleton of the limb is formed by___________ mesoderm
    a) Paraxial b) Lateral
    c) Intermediate d) Chorda
24. The paraxial mesoderm forms ____________
    a) Muscles of the limbs b) Axial skeleton
    c) Trunk muscles d) All of these
25. Germ layer origin of the nervous system
    a) Ectoderm b) Entoderm
    c) Mesoderm d) None of these
26. The somites develops from which of the following
    a) Axial mesoderm b) Paraxial mesoderm
    c) Lateral mesoderm d) Intermediate mesoderm
27. The organs of urinary system develops from
    a) Axial mesoderm b) Lateral mesoderm
    c) Intermediate mesoderm d) Paraxial mesoderm
28. In which week of gestation (mammals) primitive streak appears first
    a) First b) Second
    c) Third d) Fourth

29. Which of the following structure is believed to be primary organizer or inducer during organogenesis
    a) Somites b) Metanephric blastoma
    c) Lens placode d) Notochord
30. The heart is derived from
    a) Splanchnic mesoderm b) Somatic mesoderm
    c) Septum transversarium d) Intermediate mesoderm
31. Epithelial lining of digestive and respiratory tract, urinary bladder and urethra are derived from
    a) Ectoderm b) Mesoderm
    c) Endoderm d) Chorionic villi
32. With formation of endoderm the blastocoele is divided into
    a) Primitive gut b) Extra embryonic coelom
    c) Both of the above d) Not divided division
33. The embryonic disc occupies a position at the
    a) animal pole b) Vegetal pole
34. A cluster of tightly packed cell at the cephalic end of primitive groove is called
    a) Henson'snode or Primitive knot. b) Cephalic node
    c) Primitive groove d) Primitive streak
35. A cell layer formed between endoderm and embryonic disc is
    a) Ectoderm b) Mesoderm
    c) Endoderm d) All germ layers
36. In primitive streak, size of superficial cell layer is ---------------than other cells types
    a) Larger b) Smaller
    c) Equal d) None of the above
37. The superficial cell layer forms the ectoderm layer, which are continuous with trophoblast cells layer known as-
    a) Trophoectoderm b) Trophoderm
    c) Trophoendoderm d) Ectoderm
38. ------------------- is a rod like rostral extension of primitive node
    a) Notochord b) Hensons node
    c) Primitive streak d) None of the above
39. Notochord extends from the ______________region ventral to the developing neural tube
    a) Cranial to caudal b) Caudal to cranial
    c) Transverse d) Vertical
40. Notochord extends from the cranial to caudal region ____________to the developing neural tube
    a) Ventral b) Dorsal
    c) Medial d) Lateral

41. ---------------------------serves as inductor/precursor for the formation of head process, nervous system and formation of somites.
   a) Notochord b) Trophoderm
   c) Trophoendoderm d) None of the above
42. The neural plate was formed by folding of
   a) Neural crest cells b) Neural plate
   c) Notochord d) Primitive streak
43. Neural crest cells are formed by
   a) Ectoderm b) Mesoderm
   c) Endoderm d) All of the above
44. Neural tube gives rise to
   a) CNS b) PNS
   c) Both of the above d) None of the above
45. The PNS develops from
   a) Neural tube
   b) Neural crest cells
   c) Both the neural tube and neural crest cells
   d) None of the above
46. The developing mesoderm is arranged into -----------distinct areas
   a) One b) Two
   c) Three d) Four
47. Mesoderm adjacent to the developing neural tube forms a thickened column of cells referred to as:
   a) Lateral mesoderm b) Intermediate mesoderm
   c) Ventral mesoderm d) Paraxial mesoderm
48. ---------------------are mesodermal segmented blocks situated on either side of neural tube
   a) Somites b) Neural folds
   c) Neural plates d) All of the above
49. The first pair of somite appears in cow at ______ days post fertilization
   a) 13 b) 17
   c) 20 d) 22
50. The first pair of somite appears in sheep at ______ days post fertilization
   a) 13 b) 17
   c) 20 d) 22
51. The first pair of somite appears in pig at ______ days post fertilization
   a) 13 b) 17
   c) 20 d) 22

52. The first pair of somite appears in chicks at ______ days post fertilization
    a) 13 b) 17
    c) 20 d) 22
53. Somites first appear in head region and are added progressively towards tail
    a) True b) False
    c) None of the above d) Incomplete sentence
54. Somites first appear in _________region
    a) Head b) Tail
    c) Abdomen d) Thorax
55. During development of embryo a small cavity is formed in center of somite called as
    a) Myocoele b) Extra embryonic coelom
    c) Intra embryonic coelom d) None of the above
56. Somites, distinctively arranged into -----------separate masses of cell :
    a) Two b) Three
    c) Four d) Five
57. The cells of ventral part of somite mixed with cells of myocoele and form
    a) Sclerotome b) Dermotome
    c) Myotome d) All of the above
58. The cells of dorso lateral part of somite form
    a) Sclerotome b) Dermotome
    c) Myotome d) All of the above
59. The cells of somite at its dorso medial part are called
    a) Sclerotome b) Dermotome
    c) Myotome d) All of the above
60. Sclerotome give rise to
    a) Vertebrae b) Appendicular skeleton
    c) Axial muscle d) Skin
61. Sclerotome give rise to
    a) Ribs b) Appendicular skeleton
    c) Axial muscle d) Skin
62. Sclerotome give rise to
    a) Basilar part of sphenoid b) Appendicular skeleton
    c) Axial muscle d) Skin
63. Sclerotome give rise to
    a) Occipital bones b) Appendicular skeleton
    c) Axial muscle d) Skin
64. Dermatome give rise to
    a) Occipital bones b) Appendicular skeleton
    c) Axial muscle and Skin d) Basilar part of sphenoid

65. Myotome give rise to
a) Occipital bones
b) Appendicular skeleton
c) Axial muscle and Skin
d) Basilar part of sphenoid

66. Mesoderm lateral to the somites forms a column of cells referred to as
a) Intermediate Mesoderm
b) Lateral mesoderm
c) Dorsal mesoderm
d) Paraxial mesoderm

67. Intermediate cell mass gives rise to:
a) Occipital bones
b) Uro- genital system
c) Axial muscle and Skin
d) Basilar part of sphenoid

68. Nephrotome gives rise to:
a) Occipital bones
b) Uro- genital system
c) Axial muscle and Skin
d) Basilar part of sphenoid

69. Small cavities intraembryonic coelom are present in
a) Intermediate Mesoderm
b) Lateral plate mesoderm
c) Dorsal mesoderm
d) Paraxial mesoderm

70. The intraembryonic coelom forms the
a) Pericardial sac
b) Heart
c) Lungs
d) Stomach

71. The intraembryonic coelom forms the
a) Peritoneum
b) Heart
c) Lungs
d) stomach

72. The intraembryonic coelom forms the
a) Pleural sac
b) Heart
c) Lungs
d) stomach

73. The intraembryonic coelom forms the
a) Pericardial and Pleural sac and Peritoneum
b) Heart
c) Lungs
d) Stomach

74. The lateral plate mesoderm divides into
a) Somatopleura
b) Splanchnopleura
c) Both of the above
d) None of the above

75. Lateral and ventral body walls of the embryo except musculature and ribs are formed by
a) Somatopleura
b) Splanchnopleura
c) Both of the above
d) None of the above

76. Most of the Gatro intestinal tract located in thorax and abdomen and lungs are formed by
a) Somatopleura
b) Splanchnopleura
c) Both of the above
d) None of the above

77. A parietal layer formed from the lateral plate mesoderm after the development of intra-embryonic coelom is

a) Somatopleura b) Splanchnopleura

c) Both of the above d) None of the above

78. A visceral layer formed from the lateral plate mesoderm after the development of intra-embryonic coelom is

a) Somatopleura b) Splanchnopleura

c) Both of the above d) None of the above

79. In pig mesoderm appears at -----------days post fertilization

a) 9 b) 12

c) 15 d) 13

80. In horse mesoderm appears at -----------days post fertilization

a) 9 b) 12-14

c) 15 d) 13

81. In cow mesoderm appears at -----------days post fertilization

a) 9 b) 12

c) 15 d) 13

82. In sheep mesoderm appears at -----------days post fertilization

a) 9 b) 12

c) 15 d) 13

83. In dog mesoderm appears at -----------days post fertilization

a) 9 b) 12

c) 15-16 d) 13

84. In pig endoderm appears at -----------days post fertilization

a) 7-8 b) 12

c) 15 d) 13

85. In cow endoderm appears at -----------days post fertilization

a) 10-11 b) 12

c) 15 d) 13

86. In horse endoderm appears at -----------days post fertilization

a) 9 b) 12

c) 15 d) 13

87. In sheep endoderm appears at -----------days post fertilization

a) 10 b) 12

c) 15 d) 13

88. In dog endoderm appears at -----------days post fertilization

a) 7-8 b) 12

c) 15 d) 13

89. Number of pairs of somites develops in ox is
 a) 45 b) 54
 c) 42 d) 57
90. Number of pairs of somites develops in horse is
 a) 45 b) 54
 c) 42 d) 57
91. Number of pairs of somites develops in ovine is
 a) 45 b) 54
 c) 42 d) 57
92. Number of pairs of somites develops in porcine is
 a) 45 b) 54
 c) 42 d) 57
93. Number of pairs of somites develops in canine is
 a) 45 b) 54
 c) 55 d) 57
94. Number of pairs of somites develops in birds is
 a) 44 b) 54
 c) 42 d) 57
95. Epidermis of skin is derived from
 a) Ectoderm b) Endoderm
 c) Mesoderm d) All of the above
96. Epithelium of oral and nasal cavities are derived from
 a) Ectoderm b) Endoderm
 c) Mesoderm d) All of the above
97. Sense organs are derived from
 a) Ectoderm b) Endoderm
 c) Mesoderm d) All of the above
98. Tip and body of the tongue are derived from
 a) Ectoderm b) Endoderm
 c) Mesoderm d) All of the above
99. Blood and blood vessels are derived from
 a) Ectoderm b) Endoderm
 c) Mesoderm d) All of the above
100. Spleen is derived from
 a) Ectoderm b) Endoderm
 c) Mesoderm d) All of the above
101. Lymphnodes are derived from
 a) Ectoderm b) Endoderm
 c) Mesoderm d) All of the above

102. Root of tongue is derived from
   a) Ectoderm b) Endoderm
   c) Mesoderm d) All of the above

103. Eustachian tube is derived from
   a) Ectoderm b) Endoderm
   c) Mesoderm d) All of the above

104. Tonsil are derived from
   a) Ectoderm b) Endoderm
   c) Mesoderm d) All of the above

105. Larynx is derived from
   a) Ectoderm b) Endoderm
   c) Mesoderm d) All of the above

106. Trachea is derived from
   a) Ectoderm b) Endoderm
   c) Mesoderm d) All of the above

107. Oesophagus is derived from
   a) Ectoderm b) Endoderm
   c) Mesoderm d) All of the above

108. Prostate gland is ________________ in origin
   a) Ectodermal b) Endodermal
   c) Mesodermal d) All of the above

109. Cowper's gland is ________________ in origin
   a) Ectodermal b) Endodermal
   c) Mesodermal d) All of the above

110. Lung is ________________ in origin
   a) Ectodermal b) Endodermal
   c) Mesodermal d) All of the above

Answer Key

1	b	2	b	3	c	4	a	5	c	6	b	7	b
8	b	9	a	10	b	11	d	12	a	13	a	14	b
15	d	16	c	17	c	18	d	19	d	20	a	21	b
22	c	23	b	24	d	25	a	26	b	27	c	28	c
29	d	30	a	31	c	32	c	33	a	34	a	35	b
36	a	37	a	38	a	39	a	40	a	41	a	42	b
43	a	44	a	45	c	46	c	47	d	48	a	49	c
50	b	51	a	52	d	53	a	54	a	55	a	56	b
57	a	58	b	59	c	60	a	61	a	62	a	63	a
64	a	65	b	66	a	67	b	68	b	69	b	70	a

71	a	72	a	73	a	74	c	75	a	76	b	77	a
78	b	79	a	80	b	81	c	82	b	83	c	84	a
85	a	86	a	87	a	88	b	89	a	90	b	91	c
92	d	93	c	94	a	95	a	96	a	97	a	98	a
99	c	100	c	101	c	102	b	103	b	104	b	105	b
106	b	107	b	108	b	109	b	110	b				

8

Cellular Signalling and Genetic Functioning

Ersavadla Rajaraviteja[1] and Suvaneeth P.[2]

[1]*Department of Veterinary Anatomy, Faculty of Veterinary and Animal Sciences, Institute of Agricultural Sciences, Rajiv Gandhi South Campus, Banaras Hindu University, Barkachha, Mirzapur-231001*

[2]*Department of Veterinary Pathology, Faculty of Veterinary and Animal Sciences, Institute of Agricultural Sciences, Rajiv Gandhi South Campus, Banaras Hindu University, Barkachha, Mirzapur-231001*

Introduction

Embryogenesis begins with the fertilization of the oocyte by the sperm, leading to the formation of a zygote. This single cell undergoes a series of highly regulated mitotic divisions known as cleavage, forming a multicellular structure called the blastocyst. As the blastocyst implants in the uterine wall, the cells continue to divide and differentiate into the three primary germ layers: the ectoderm, mesoderm, and endoderm. Each of these layers gives rise to specific tissues and organs, controlled by genetic instructions and cellular signalling mechanisms.One of the most critical aspects of embryogenesis is the intricate interplay of cellular signalling pathways and genetic mechanisms, which regulate the precise growth and differentiation of cells into tissues and organs. Understanding these mechanisms not only helps in comprehending normal embryonic development but also in diagnosing and treating developmental disorders in veterinary practice.

Cellular Signalling in Embryonic Development

Cellular signalling is a fundamental process in embryogenesis that ensures cells communicate with each other to perform specific tasks. The coordination of cell proliferation, differentiation, migration, and apoptosis (programmed cell death) is essential for the proper formation of tissues and organs.

Types of cell signalling

1. **Short range signalling:** It involves communication within a cell as well as between nearby cells. This includes:
   a) **Paracrine signalling:** where a cell releases signals that affect neighbouring cells.
   b) **Autocrine signalling:** where a cell sends signals to itself, affecting its own behaviour.

   c) **Contact-dependent signalling:** where cells communicate through direct physical contact with each other.

2. **Long range signalling:** It involves communication between cells located at a distance from each other. This includes:
   a) **Synaptic signalling:** where neurons transmit signals across long distances through specialized structures called synapses.
   b) **Endocrine signalling:** where hormones are released into the bloodstream and travel to distant target cells throughout the body.

Several key signalling pathways are involved in these processes, including:

1. Wnt Signalling Pathway

The Wnt signalling pathway plays a crucial role in cell fate determination, tissue patterning, and the regulation of cell proliferation. During early embryonic development, Wnt signals are involved in axis formation, which determines the body's anterior-posterior orientation. Misregulation of the Wnt pathway can result in developmental abnormalities such as neural tube defects and skeletal malformations.

There are two main Wnt signalling cascades: the canonical and non-canonical pathways. The canonical pathway involves β-catenin, which, when activated by Wnt ligands, translocates to the nucleus to modulate gene expression. The non-canonical pathway, on the other hand, regulates cell movement and polarity independent of β-catenin.

2. Hedgehog Signalling Pathway

The Hedgehog (Hh) pathway is critical for the patterning of various tissues, including the brain, limbs, and gastrointestinal tract. Sonic Hedgehog (Shh) is the most widely studied ligand of this pathway in vertebrates. Shh signalling guides the formation of the neural tube and somites, which are precursors to the vertebrae and associated muscle groups.

During limb development, Shh is expressed in the zone of polarizing activity (ZPA)) and establishes the anterior-posterior axis, ensuring proper limb formation. Mutations in components of the Hedgehog pathway can lead to congenital malformations such as cyclopia (single-eyed embryo) or polydactyly (extra digits).

3. Notch Signalling Pathway

The Notch pathway is involved in cell-cell communication and influences cell fate decisions, proliferation, and apoptosis. It is especially important in maintaining a balance between stem cell proliferation and differentiation. In early embryonic development, Notch signalling regulates the differentiation of neural progenitor cells into neurons, astrocytes, and oligodendrocytes. Furthermore, the Notch pathway is involved in somite formation, which is critical for musculoskeletal development.

4. Fibroblast Growth Factor (FGF) Signalling

FGFs are a family of growth factors that play essential roles in cell proliferation, differentiation, and migration. The FGF signalling pathway is involved in various aspects of embryogenesis, including limb and organ development, angiogenesis (formation of blood vessels), and wound healing. FGF signalling is crucial for the induction of mesoderm and the development of limbs and lungs. Aberrations in FGF signalling are associated with skeletal dysplasia's and craniosynostosis (premature fusion of skull bones).

5. Bone Morphogenetic Protein (BMP) Signalling

BMPs, members of the transforming growth factor-beta (TGF-β) superfamily, are important regulators of cell growth, differentiation, and apoptosis. During embryonic development, BMP signalling controls the formation of bones, cartilage, and the nervous system. BMPs are involved in dorsal-ventral axis formation and organogenesis, particularly in the heart, kidneys, and lungs. Dysregulation of BMP signalling can result in congenital malformations such as cleft palate and cardiovascular defects.

Genetic Functioning in Embryogenesis

While cellular signalling provides the external cues for development, the genetic code within each cell dictates the specific proteins that will be expressed, leading to the specialization of cells into different tissue types. Genetic functioning during embryonic development involves gene expression, transcription factors, epigenetic regulation, and non-coding RNAs, all of which contribute to the control of developmental processes.

1. Homeobox (Hox) Genes

Hox genes are a subset of homeotic genes that regulate the body plan of an embryo along the head-to-tail axis. They are responsible for determining the identity and position of structures such as limbs, vertebrae, and organs. The precise expression of Hox genes in specific regions of the embryo ensures that body parts form in the correct locations. For example, mutations in Hox genes can lead to homeotic transformations, where one body part is replaced by another, such as an extra set of ribs or abnormal limb positioning.

2. Epigenetic Regulation

Epigenetic mechanisms, including DNA methylation, histone modifications, and chromatin remodeling, play a crucial role in regulating gene expression during embryogenesis. These modifications do not alter the DNA sequence but instead influence the accessibility of genes to transcription factors, thereby controlling whether specific genes are activated or silenced. Epigenetic regulation ensures that different cell types express only the genes necessary for their function, allowing for the differentiation of stem cells into specialized cells such as neurons, muscle cells, and hepatocytes.

3. Transcription Factors

Transcription factors are proteins that bind to specific DNA sequences to regulate gene expression. During embryonic development, transcription factors such as Oct4, Sox2, and Nanog maintain the pluripotency of embryonic stem cells, allowing them to differentiate into any cell type. As development progresses, other transcription factors, including Pax6, MyoD, and GATA4, drive the differentiation of specific cell lineages, such as the nervous system, muscle, and cardiac tissue, respectively.

4. Non-coding RNAs

Non-coding RNAs, including microRNAs (miRNAs) and long non-coding RNAs (lncRNAs), are involved in post-transcriptional regulation of gene expression during embryogenesis. miRNAs bind to messenger RNAs (mRNAs) to inhibit their translation or promote their degradation, thereby fine-tuning protein expression levels. lncRNAs, on the other hand, can regulate gene expression by interacting with chromatin, transcription factors, or mRNAs. Dysregulation of non-coding RNAs has been linked to various developmental disorders and congenital anomalies.

Clinical Relevance in Veterinary Medicine

A thorough understanding of cellular signalling and genetic functioning in embryology is essential for veterinarians, especially in the diagnosis and treatment of congenital disorders. Many developmental defects in animals, such as cleft palate, limb malformations, and neural tube defects, can be traced back to disruptions in these signalling pathways and genetic mechanisms.

Moreover, advances in genetic engineering and stem cell therapy hold promise for treating congenital defects in animals. For instance, gene editing techniques such as CRISPR-Cas9 can potentially correct mutations responsible for genetic disorders, while stem cell therapies can regenerate damaged tissues and organs.

Conclusion

Veterinary embryology is a field that encompasses the coordinated actions of cellular signalling pathways and genetic mechanisms, which are essential for the proper development of an organism. Disruptions in these processes can lead to congenital abnormalities and developmental disorders. As our understanding of embryonic signalling and genetic functioning continues to grow, so too will our ability to diagnose, prevent, and treat developmental defects in veterinary medicine, ultimately improving animal health and well-being.

Multiple Choice Questions

1. Which type of cellular signaling involves a cell responding to signals it secretes itself ?

   a) Autocrine signaling b) Paracrine signaling
   c) Endocrine signaling d) Juxtacrinesignaling

2. What is the role of gap junctions in cellular communication?

   a) Allow direct cell-to-cell signaling b) Transmit endocrine signals
   c) Prevent cells from communicating d) Facilitate paracrine signaling

3. Which signaling pathway is critical for embryonic development and regulates cell fate decisions?

   a) Wntsignaling b) Ras/MAPK signaling
   c) JAK/STAT signaling d) Hedgehog signaling

4. Which family of proteins is involved in the regulation of programmed cell death (apoptosis) during embryogenesis?

   a) Cyclins b) Caspases
   c) Integrins d) G proteins

5. Sonic hedgehog (Shh) is an important signaling molecule during which process of embryonic development?

   a) Limb patterning b) Axon guidance
   c) Cell division d) Apoptosis

6. Which signaling molecule is known for its role in establishing the dorsal-ventral axis during embryogenesis?
   a) Sonic hedgehog (Shh)
   b) Wnt
   c) Bone morphogenetic protein (BMP)
   d) Fibroblast growth factor (FGF)
7. Which gene family is responsible for anterior-posterior body patterning during embryonic development?
   a) HOX genes
   b) Ras genes
   c) G-protein coupled receptors
   d) Notch genes
8. Which type of cell signaling is involved when a signal molecule is released and affects only nearby cells?
   a) Paracrine signaling
   b) Autocrine signaling
   c) Endocrine signaling
   d) Synaptic signaling
9. The Notch signaling pathway is important for which embryonic process?
   a) Cell differentiation
   b) Cell proliferation
   c) Limb formation
   d) Axon guidance
10. Which protein is the receptor in the Wntsignaling pathway?
    a) Smoothened
    b) Patched
    c) Frizzled
    d) Gli
11. Which embryonic layer gives rise to the nervous system and skin?
    a) Endoderm
    b) Mesoderm
    c) Ectoderm
    d) Trophoblast
12. Which signaling pathway involves the activation of Smad proteins in response to ligand binding?
    a) Wnt pathway
    b) TGF-β (Transforming growth factor-beta pathway)
    c) Hedgehog pathway
    d) JAK/STAT pathway
13. Which molecule is central to the control of the cell cycle and its checkpoints during embryogenesis?
    a) p53
    b) Cyclins
    c) Integrins
    d) Tubulins
14. What is the role of FGF (fibroblast growth factor) signaling in embryonic development?
    a) Regulation of cell proliferation and differentiation
    b) Induction of apoptosis
    c) DNA replication
    d) Nutrient transport
15. Which family of signaling molecules plays a crucial role in limb formation?
    a) Wnt
    b) FGF
    c) Notch
    d) Ras

16. Which protein is essential in the Ras/MAPK signaling pathway for transmitting signals from membrane receptors to the nucleus?
    a) Ras
    b) Smad
    c) Gli
    d) Notch
17. Which signaling mechanism involves cells in direct contact, often using proteins embedded in the plasma membrane?
    a) Endocrine signaling
    b) Paracrine signaling
    c) Juxtacrinesignaling
    d) Synaptic signaling
18. Which signaling pathway is critical in neural tube closure during embryogenesis?
    a) Sonic hedgehog pathway
    b) Wnt pathway
    c) FGF pathway
    d) Notch pathway
19. Which type of signaling is essential for the regulation of vascular development in embryos?
    a) VEGF (vascular endothelial growth factor) signaling
    b) Wntsignaling
    c) BMP signaling
    d) Ras/MAPK signaling
20. Which signaling molecule is primarily involved in neural crest cell migration during embryogenesis?
    a) Ephrins
    b) BMP
    c) Notch
    d) Retinoic acid
21. What is the role of HOX genes in embryonic development?
    a) DNA replication
    b) Cell division control
    c) Segmental identity along the anterior-posterior axis
    d) Programmed cell death
22. Which of the following is a key downstream effector in the JAK/STAT signaling pathway?
    a) Smad
    b) STAT
    c) Ras
    d) Gli
23. The Wnt/β-catenin signaling pathway is best known for its role in which embryonic process?
    a) Regulation of cell proliferation and differentiation
    b) Inducing apoptosis
    c) Cell motility
    d) DNA replication
24. Which structure releases signaling molecules to establish the left-right axis during early embryonic development?
    a) Notochord
    b) Neural tube
    c) Primitive node (Hensen's node)
    d) Somites

25. The TGF-β superfamily includes which signaling molecules important for embryonic patterning?

a) BMPs (Bone morphogenetic proteins) b) Wnts
c) Hedgehog proteins d) FGF proteins

26. Which gene regulatory process is central to epigenetic changes during embryogenesis?

a) DNA methylation b) RNA transcription
c) Protein translation d) Chromatin condensation

27. Notch signaling is important for which of the following processes in embryonic development?

a) Limb patterning b) Apoptosis
c) Cell fate determination d) Vascular formation

28. Which protein is a critical transcription factor in the Sonic hedgehog (Shh) signaling pathway?

a) Gli b) STAT
c) Smad d) Wnt

29. What is the role of retinoic acid (RA) in embryonic development?

a) Regulates HOX gene expression b) Controls DNA replication
c) Stimulates cell proliferation d) Induces apoptosis

30. Which gene is involved in the regulation of cell proliferation and apoptosis and is often referred to as the "guardian of the genome"?

a) p53 b) Ras
c) Gli d) BMP

31. Which embryonic signaling pathway is activated by binding of ligands to receptor tyrosine kinases (RTKs)?

a) Ras/MAPK signaling pathway b) Notch signaling pathway
c) Wntsignaling pathway d) Hedgehog signaling pathway

32. Which signaling pathway is crucial for somite formation during early embryogenesis?

a) Notch signaling pathway b) Wntsignaling pathway
c) BMP signaling pathway d) Ras/MAPK signaling pathway

33. Apoptosis is tightly regulated during development to remove unneeded cells. Which pathway is central to the intrinsic apoptosis mechanism?

a) Ras/MAPK signaling pathway
b) Caspase pathway
c) JAK/STAT pathway
d) Wnt/β-catenin signaling pathway

34. Which of the following molecules regulates mesoderm patterning during gastrulation?

a) Nodal b) BMP
c) FGF d) Shh

35. The Wntsignaling pathway is primarily involved in which of the following processes?
    a) Regulating cell proliferation and migration
    b) Triggering apoptosis
    c) Inducing neural crest cell migration
    d) Controlling DNA replication

36. What is the function of cadherins in embryogenesis?
    a) Facilitate cell adhesion
    b) Induce apoptosis
    c) Trigger DNA replication
    d) Initiate signal transduction

37. Which signaling molecule is essential for the induction of lens formation in vertebrates?
    a) FGF
    b) Shh
    c) BMP
    d) Notch

38. Which cellular structure plays a key role in organizing the body axes during early vertebrate embryogenesis?
    a) Notochord
    b) Primitive streak
    c) Neural crest
    d) Somites

39. Which embryonic signaling pathway is responsible for vascular remodeling and angiogenesis?
    a) VEGF signaling pathway
    b) Wnt/β-catenin signaling pathway
    c) Shh signaling pathway
    d) Ras/MAPK signaling pathway

40. Which structure releases morphogens like Sonic hedgehog (Shh) that are involved in patterning the developing embryo?
    a) Notochord
    b) Neural crest
    c) Somites
    d) Neural tube

41. Which transcription factor is central to the regulation of limb development and differentiation?
    a) Gli
    b) HOX genes
    c) Pax6
    d) STAT

42. Which type of cellular signaling involves the release of hormones into the bloodstream to reach distant target cells?
    a) Endocrine signaling
    b) Paracrine signaling
    c) Autocrine signaling
    d) Synaptic signaling

43. Which molecule is involved in the control of the cell cycle and serves as a tumor suppressor in developing tissues?
    a) p53
    b) Ras
    c) FGF
    d) Gli

44. What is the role of the TGF-β signaling pathway in embryogenesis?
   a) Controls cell growth, proliferation, and differentiation
   b) Induces neural crest migration
   c) Activates apoptosis in limb development
   d) Stimulates DNA replication

45. Which signaling molecule is primarily responsible for posterior limb development during embryogenesis?
   a) Sonic hedgehog (Shh) b) BMP
   c) FGF d) Wnt

46. Which process during embryogenesis involves the formation of distinct layers of cells, such as the ectoderm, mesoderm, and endoderm?
   a) Gastrulation b) Neurulation
   c) Apoptosis d) Induction

47. Which signaling pathway regulates the fate of neural progenitor cells during brain development?
   a) Notch signaling pathway b) FGF signaling pathway
   c) Hedgehog signaling pathway d) JAK/STAT signaling pathway

48. Which molecule is involved in the regulation of the cell cycle by binding to and activating cyclin-dependent kinases (CDKs)?
   a) Cyclins b) Gli proteins
   c) Ras proteins d) Wnt proteins

49. What is the main role of Smad proteins in embryonic development?
   a) Mediate signaling in the TGF-β pathway
   b) Trigger apoptosis in neurons
   c) Activate the Wntsignaling pathway
   d) Control angiogenesis

50. Which gene family is essential for patterning the vertebrate body along the anterior-posterior axis?
   a) HOX genes b) Pax genes
   c) Myc genes d) STAT genes

51. What role do microRNAs (miRNAs) play during embryonic development?
   a) Regulate gene expression post-transcriptionally
   b) Control cell adhesion
   c) Facilitate protein folding
   d) Induce apoptosis

52. The activation of which signaling pathway is essential for the formation of somites during vertebrate development?
   a) Notch signaling pathway b) Ras/MAPK signaling pathway
   c) Hedgehog signaling pathway d) VEGF signaling pathway

53. Which protein functions as a tumor suppressor and is essential in preventing uncontrolled cell growth during development?

a) p53 b) Ras

c) Cyclin D d) Pax6

54. Which signaling pathway regulates the maintenance and differentiation of stem cells in embryonic tissues?

a) Wntsignaling pathway b) TGF-β signaling pathway

c) Notch signaling pathway d) Ras/MAPK signaling pathway

55. Which transcription factor is essential for eye development in vertebrates?

a) Pax6 b) HOX genes

c) Gli proteins d) Smad proteins

56. Which of the following processes is regulated by Wntsignaling during vertebrate embryogenesis?

a) Axis formation and cell polarity b) Apoptosis in the neural tube

c) Neural crest migration d) Muscle differentiation

57. What is the role of the retinoic acid (RA)) signaling pathway during development?

a) Regulates patterning of the anterior-posterior axis

b) Triggers apoptosis in neural cells

c) Induces neural crest cell formation

d) Stimulates limb bud growth

58. The activation of which pathway is essential for the development of the anterior-posterior axis in embryos?

a) Wntsignaling pathway b) Notch signaling pathway

c) BMP signaling pathway d) Ras/MAPK signaling pathway

59. Which signaling pathway involves the phosphorylation and activation of STAT proteins?

a) JAK/STAT signaling pathway b) Hedgehog signaling pathway

c) TGF-β signaling pathway d) Wntsignaling pathway

60. Which molecule serves as a ligand in the Hedgehog signaling pathway and is crucial for vertebrate limb development?

a) Sonic hedgehog (Shh) b) Wnt

c) BMP d) FGF

61. Which protein is activated in the Wnt/β-catenin pathway and plays a role in transcriptional regulation during development?

a) β-catenin b) Gli

c) Cyclin D d) Pax6

62. Which signaling pathway is activated by binding of extracellular matrix proteins to integrins during embryogenesis?
   a) FAK (Focal adhesion kinase) signaling pathway
   b) Notch signaling pathway
   c) Hedgehog signaling pathway
   d) JAK/STAT signaling pathway

63. What is the role of BMP signaling in embryonic development?
   a) Establishes the dorsal-ventral axis b) Regulates eye formation
   c) Controls limb bud growth d) Activates neural crest migration

64. The TGF-β signaling pathway plays a major role in which embryonic processes?
   a) Cell proliferation and differentiation b) Cell migration and motility
   c) Apoptosis and cell deathd) DNA replication and transcription

65. Which family of signaling molecules is involved in establishing the left-right body axis in vertebrates?
   a) Nodal proteins b) BMP proteins
   c) Wnt proteins d) Shh proteins

66. Which structure is responsible for signaling the development of the neural tube in early vertebrate embryos?
   a) Notochord b) Primitive streak
   c) Neural crest d) Somites

67. Which signaling pathway is primarily involved in the control of neural differentiation during brain development?
   a) Notch signaling pathway b) Ras/MAPK signaling pathway
   c) TGF-β signaling pathway d) JAK/STAT signaling pathway

68. Which protein family is central to establishing polarity and differentiation of epithelial cells during embryogenesis?
   a) Cadherins b) Integrins
   c) Pax proteins d) Cyclins

69. Which signaling pathway plays a key role in the development of the respiratory system during vertebrate embryogenesis?
   a) FGF signaling pathway b) Notch signaling pathway
   c) Wntsignaling pathway d) Hedgehog signaling pathway

70. Which pathway is responsible for regulating blood vessel formation during development?
   a) VEGF signaling pathway b) TGF-β signaling pathway
   c) Wntsignaling pathway d) Hedgehog signaling pathway

71. Which signaling molecule induces the formation of neural crest cells during vertebrate embryogenesis?
   a) BMP b) FGF
   c) Wnt d) Shh

72. Which gene is involved in the segmentation and identity of specific regions along the vertebrate anterior-posterior axis?

a) HOX genes
b) Pax genes
c) Gli genes
d) Smad genes

73. Which signaling pathway is activated in response to mechanical stress during embryogenesis?

a) FAK (Focal adhesion kinase) signaling pathway
b) TGF-β signaling pathway
c) Ras/MAPK signaling pathway
d) JAK/STAT signaling pathway

74. Which transcription factor is crucial for neural crest development and differentiation in vertebrates?

a) Pax3
b) HOX genes
c) STAT
d) Cyclins

75. Which signaling pathway is critical for establishing tissue polarity during embryogenesis?

a) Wnt/β-catenin signaling pathway
b) TGF-β signaling pathway
c) Hedgehog signaling pathway
d) Ras/MAPK signaling pathway

76. Which protein family plays a role in the control of cell migration during embryogenesis by binding to extracellular matrix components?

a) Integrins
b) Cyclins
c) Pax proteins
d) Gli proteins

77. Which signaling molecule is involved in the regulation of the left-right body axis and heart development?

a) Nodal
b) Wnt
c) FGF
d) Pax6

78. What is the role of retinoic acid (RA) during embryonic development?

a) Regulates HOX gene expression
b) Controls DNA replication
c) Stimulates apoptosis
d) Induces muscle differentiation

79. Which molecule is critical for maintaining stem cell populations during vertebrate development?

a) Wnt
b) Shh
c) FGF
d) Pax6

80. The JAK/STAT signaling pathway is essential in regulating which developmental processes?

a) Immune cell differentiation and proliferation
b) Neural crest migration
c) Limb patterning
d) Eye development

81. Which signaling pathway is involved in the regulation of cartilage and bone formation during embryonic development?
   a) BMP signaling pathway b) Notch signaling pathway
   c) Wntsignaling pathway d) Hedgehog signaling pathway

82. Which protein functions as a tumor suppressor and is essential in controlling cell cycle checkpoints during development?
   a) p53 b) Ras
   c) Cyclin B d) Gli

83. Which signaling molecule is crucial for inducing the formation of mesoderm during early vertebrate development?
   a) Nodal b) BMP
   c) FGF d) Shh

84. What is the role of cadherins in embryonic development?
   a) Facilitate cell-cell adhesion b) Stimulate cell division
   c) Activate signal transduction pathways d) Control apoptosis

85. Which signaling pathway is involved in the establishment of body segments in vertebrates?
   a) Notch signaling pathway b) Ras/MAPK signaling pathway
   c) JAK/STAT signaling pathway d) TGF-β signaling pathway

86. Which signaling molecule is primarily involved in angiogenesis and blood vessel formation during development?
   a) VEGF b) FGF
   c) BMP d) Wnt

87. Which transcription factor plays a key role in eye development in vertebrates?
   a) Pax6 b) HOX genes
   c) STAT d) Cyclin D

88. Which pathway is involved in the regulation of apoptosis during limb formation?
   a) BMP signaling pathway b) Ras/MAPK signaling pathway
   c) Notch signaling pathway d) JAK/STAT signaling pathway

89. Which protein is responsible for transmitting signals in the Hedgehog signaling pathway?
   a) Smoothened b) STAT
   c) Ras d) Cyclin B

90. Which signaling pathway is critical for regulating proliferation and differentiation of hematopoietic stem cells?
   a) JAK/STAT signaling pathway b) Wntsignaling pathway
   c) BMP signaling pathway d) FGF signaling pathway

91. Which of the following is essential for cell-cell communication during early embryogenesis?
   a) Gap junctions b) Integrins
   c) Cyclins d) Pax proteins

92. Which signaling pathway is involved in the differentiation of muscle cells during vertebrate development?
    a) Wnt/β-catenin signaling pathway   b) TGF-β signaling pathway
    c) Notch signaling pathway   d) Ras/MAPK signaling pathway

93. What role does FGF signaling play in vertebrate limb development?
    a) Controls limb bud outgrowth and patterning
    b) Regulates cell polarity and adhesion
    c) Induces neural crest cell differentiation
    d) Promotes apoptosis in the neural tube

94. Which family of proteins mediates the degradation of β-catenin in the absence of Wntsignaling?
    a) APC (Adenomatous polyposis coli) proteins
    b) Gli proteins
    c) Smad proteins
    d) Cyclin D proteins

95. Which signaling pathway is activated during the development of the heart and vasculature in vertebrates?
    a) VEGF signaling pathway   b) Ras/MAPK signaling pathway
    c) JAK/STAT signaling pathway   d) Notch signaling pathway

96. Which signaling molecule is crucial for specifying motor neuron identity in the developing spinal cord?
    a) Sonic hedgehog (Shh)   b) FGF
    c) BMP   d) Notch

97. What is the role of FAK (Focal adhesion kinase) in embryogenesis?
    a) Transmits signals from integrins to regulate cell migration and adhesion
    b) Activates apoptosis in limb formation
    c) Controls neural crest migration
    d) Induces muscle differentiation

98. Which signaling molecule is required for dorsal-ventral patterning in vertebrate embryos?
    a) BMP   b) FGF
    c) Shh   d) Wnt

99. Which of the following is crucial for establishing tissue polarity and directing cell movement during gastrulation?
    a) Wntsignaling pathway   b) FGF signaling pathway
    c) TGF-β signaling pathway   d) Notch signaling pathway

100. Which signaling pathway is central to the maintenance and self-renewal of stem cells in embryonic tissues?
    a) Wntsignaling pathway   b) TGF-β signaling pathway
    c) Notch signaling pathway   d) Ras/MAPK signaling pathway

Answer Key

1	a	2	a	3	d	4	b	5	a	6	c	7	a
8	a	9	a	10	c	11	c	12	b	13	b	14	a
15	b	16	a	17	c	18	a	19	a	20	a	21	c
22	b	23	a	24	c	25	a	26	a	27	c	28	a
29	a	30	a	31	a	32	a	33	b	34	a	35	a
36	a	37	a	38	b	39	a	40	a	41	b	42	a
43	a	44	a	45	a	46	a	47	a	48	a	49	a
50	a	51	a	52	a	53	a	54	a	55	a	56	a
57	a	58	a	59	a	60	a	61	a	62	a	63	a
64	a	65	a	66	a	67	a	68	a	69	a	70	a
71	a	72	a	73	a	74	a	75	a	76	a	77	a
78	a	79	a	80	a	81	a	82	a	83	a	84	a
85	a	86	a	87	a	88	a	89	a	90	a	91	a
92	a	93	a	94	a	95	a	96	a	97	a	98	a
99	a	100	a										

9

Stem Cells

Dayanidhi Jena[1], Sabita Behera[2], Sakshi[3], Utkarsh K. Tripathi[1] and Kruti D. Mandal[1]

[1]Faculty of Veterinary and Animal Sciences, Institute of Agricultural Sciences Banaras Hindu University, Mirzapur, U.P.

[2]Division of Bacteriology and Mycology, Indian Veterinary Research Institute Bareilly, U.P.

[3]Division of Medicine, Indian Veterinary Research Institute, Bareilly, U.P.

Introduction

Stem cells are the undifferentiated cells of the body which have inherent capacity to differentiate and proliferate into any cell type under programmed command.

These cells perpetuate themselves through self-renewal by programmed pathways to give rise to new adult cells (Remya *et al.,* 2014). According to plasticity, the stem cells are categorised into totipotent, pluripotent, multipotent and unipotent. Broadly they can also be classified as embryonic stem cells and adult somatic stem cells. Totipotent stem cells are those which can give rise to all types of cells along with placental membranes whereas pluripotent stem cells give rise to all cell types except placental membranes. The multipotent set of stem cells can give rise to more than one cell type and unipotent ones can differentiate into only one type of cells. Mesenchymal stem cells (MSCs), which fall under the multipotent stem cells category, have the multilineage potential to differentiate into many mesenchymal lineages like osteocytes, chondrocytes, adipocytes etc. (Kim *et. al.*, 2013).

They can be easily isolated from the adipose tissues, bone marrows, muscles, liver, umbilical cords, lungs etc. and can be easily proliferated *in vitro*. MSCs were first identified from the bone marrow in a pioneering study by Fredenstein *et al* (1976) who isolated the bone forming progenitor cells from rat bone marrow. Although the MSCs represent very small fraction of 0.001-0.01% of total nucleated marrow cells, they can be isolated and differentiated into multiple lineages under defined culture conditions. They are generally isolated from iliac crest, tibial and femoral marrow compartments along with thoracic and lumbar spine in large animals.

Stem cells have been used for cellular therapy and tissue engineering for quite a period of time owing to their regeneration potential. They are unspecialized cells with the ability to renew themselves for long periods without significant changes in their general properties. These cells under the influence of appropriate signals can differentiate into specialized cells with a phenotype distinct from that of the precursor (Kim *et al*., 2013). It may be that stem cells in adult tissues are reservoirs of reparative cells, ready to mobilize and differentiate in response to wound signals or disease conditions (Barry and Morphy, 2004). They have been used for many diseases and grafting of organs after the discovery of their healing potential (Blanc *et al.*, 2018). Mesenchymal stem cells, which are a type of multipotent stem cells, were first reported by Friedenstein *et al.* (1976) in rat bone marrow. They demonstrated the presence of non-hematopoietic mesenchymal precursor cells in the bone marrow, which could differentiate into cartilage or bone. These foci of cultured cells were named as colony forming unit-fibroblast (CFU-F). The term, mesenchyme, is derived from the Greek meaning "middle" (meso) "infusion" and refers to the ability of mesenchymatous cells to spread and migrate in early embryonic development between the ectodermal and endodermal layers. This characteristic migratory, space-filling ability is the key element of all wound repair in adult organisms involving mesenchymal cells in skin (dermis), bone (periosteum), or muscle (perimysium). Apart from that they have regeneration property, multipotent activity and culturally expandable *in vitro* with exceptional genomic stability marking its importance in cell therapy and regenerative medicine. These cells are also reported to possess immunomodulatory properties that enable them to escape the host immune response. When delivered systemically these cells home to the site of injury and help in regeneration of the tissue. Currently, MSCs are considered prospective therapeutic stem cells for treatment of various conditions like myocardial disease, cerebral infarction, spinal cord injury, liver damage, bone fracture, wound damaged ligament and joint injuries. MSCs have also shown better therapeutic outcomes for cell and gene-based therapies in number of congenital and degenerative diseases.

Multiple Choice Questions

1. What is the primary role of stem cells in embryonic development?
   a) Differentiation into specialized cell types
   b) Production of growth factors
   c) Maintenance of homeostasis
   d) None of the above
2. Which type of stem cells are responsible for forming the three primary germ layers during embryogenesis?
   a) Embryonic stem cells
   b) Mesenchymal stem cells
   c) Induced pluripotent stem cells
   d) Adult stem cells
3. Which stage of embryonic development involves the formation of a blastocyst containing pluripotent stem cells?
   a) Gastrulation
   b) Cleavage
   c) Blastulation
   d) Fertilization
4. What is the term for stem cells derived from the inner cell mass of a blastocyst?
   a) Adult stem cells
   b) Embryonic stem cells
   c) Multipotent stem cells
   d) Hematopoietic stem cells
5. Which type of stem cells are used for therapeutic purposes due to their multipotency ability?
   a) Adult stem cells
   b) Embryonic stem cells
   c) Induced pluripotent stem cell
   d) Mesenchymal stem cells

6. During which phase of embryogenesis do stem cells start to differentiate into specific cell lineages?
   a) Blastulation
   b) Cleavage
   c) Gastrulation
   d) Fertilization

7. What is the main ethical concern surrounding the use of embryonic stem cells in research and therapy?
   a) Limited availability
   b) Potential for tumor formation
   c) Destruction of embryos
   d) Risk of immune rejection

8. Which of the following statements about induced pluripotent stem cells (iPSCs) is true?
   a) They are derived from adult stem cells.
   b) They have limited potential for differentiation.
   c) They are obtained from blastocysts.
   d) They are reprogrammed from adult cells to an embryonic-like state.

9. What is the significance of stem cells in developmental biology and regenerative medicine?
   a) They offer potential treatments for various diseases.
   b) They allow for the study of early embryonic development.
   c) They provide insights into cellular differentiation.
   d) All of the above

10. What is the primary role of embryonic stem cells during embryonic development?
    a) Formation of extraembryonic membranes
    b) Contribution to the formation of the embryo proper
    c) Induction of placental development
    d) Formation of neural tube

11. Which cells have the potential to develop into all cell types, including extraembryonic tissues?
    a) Embryonic stem cells
    b) Totipotent cells
    c) Adult stem cells
    d) Induced pluripotent stem cells

12. Which stage of embryonic development involves the differentiation of cells into ectoderm, mesoderm, and endoderm?
    a) Blastocyst stage
    b) Cleavage stage
    c) Gastrulation
    d) Implantation

13. How are induced pluripotent stem cells typically generated in the laboratory?
    a) From embryonic stem cells
    b) By reprogramming adult somatic cells
    c) From neural stem cells
    d) Through differentiation of germ cells

14. During which phase of embryonic development do stem cells play a crucial role in the formation of organs and organ systems?
    a) Cleavage stage
    b) Blastocyst stage
    c) Gastrulation
    d) Fertilization stage
15. What is the primary role of trophoblast cells in early embryonic development?
    a) Formation of the embryonic disc
    b) Contribution to the inner cell mass
    c) Formation of the placenta
    d) Differentiation into endoderm
16. Which type of cells give rise to gametes in the embryo?
    a) Embryonic stem cells
    b) Induced pluripotent stem cells
    c) Embryonic germ cells
    d) Adult stem cells
17. Which stem cells contribute to the formation of insulin-producing β cells in the pancreas?
    a) Embryonic stem cells
    b) Induced pluripotent stem cells
    c) Mesenchymal stem cells
    d) Pancreatic progenitor cells
18. What is a common method used to induce stem cell differentiation in the laboratory?
    a) Exposing stem cells to extreme temperatures.
    b) Co-culture with differentiated cells.
    c) Using electromagnetic radiation.
    d) Using anti-inflammatory drugs
19. Why is understanding stem cell differentiation important?
    a) It helps in cloning animals.
    b) It has applications in regenerative medicine.
    c) It is useful in agriculture.
    d) All of the above.
20. What are some challenges in controlling stem cell differentiation?
    a) Ensuring consistent direction towards desired lineages.
    b) Avoiding teratoma formation.
    c) Mimicking natural developmental cues.
    d) All of the above
21. What defines a stem cell?
    a) A cell that can divide and differentiate into various specialized cell types
    b) A cell that only produces red blood cells
    c) A cell that cannot replicate
    d) A cell that is already fully specialized

22. What is the unique property of pluripotent stem cells?
    a) They can only form muscle cells
    b) They can develop into any cell type in the body
    c) They are limited to forming blood cells
    d) They can only replicate a limited number of times
23. Which characteristic is specific to multipotent stem cells?
    a) They can become any cell type in the body
    b) They can form cell types within a specific lineage or tissue
    c) They are incapable of self-renewal
    d) They exist only in embryos
24. What does "self-renewal" mean in relation to stem cells?
    a) The ability to become any cell type
    b) The capacity to undergo continuous cell division while maintaining an undifferentiated state
    c) The transformation into differentiated cells
    d) The capacity to form only blood cells
25. What distinguishes totipotent stem cells from other types?
    a) They can form any cell type and the extraembryonic tissues necessary for embryonic development
    b) They are limited to forming neural cells
    c) They can only form muscle cells
    d) They are restricted to adult tissues
26. Which of the following best describes a pluripotent stem cell?
    a) A cell that can differentiate into any cell type in the body
    b) A cell that can only become muscle cells
    c) A cell that can replicate only a few times
    d) A cell that is already fully differentiated
27. What is the primary characteristic of multipotent stem cells?
    a) They can become any type of cell
    b) They can only become cell types within a certain tissue or organ
    c) They are permanently inactive
    d) They exist only in embryos
28. Which of the following is a defining feature of totipotent stem cells?
    a) Ability to form any cell type and extraembryonic tissues
    b) Restricted to forming blood cells only
    c) Limited to creating skin cells
    d) Capable of differentiating only into neural cells

29. What does the term "self-renewal" refer to in the context of stem cells?
    a) The process of forming specialized cells
    b) The ability to replicate and maintain an undifferentiated state
    c) The transformation into cancer cells
    d) The ability to migrate throughout the body
30. Which statement accurately defines induced pluripotent stem cells (iPSCs)?
    a) Naturally occurring stem cells found in bone marrow
    b) Stem cells derived from reprogrammed adult cells
    c) Stem cells limited to forming blood cells
    d) Cells that spontaneously turn into stem cells
31. Where are mesenchymal stem cells commonly harvested from?
    a) Blood b) Liver
    c) Bone marrow d) Pancreas
32. Embryonic stem cells are typically obtained from?
    a) Adult bone marrow b) Umbilical cord
    c) Blastocyst stage embryos d) Skin biopsies
33. What is the primary goal of using stem cells in veterinary gynecology?
    a) To enhance animal growth
    b) To improve reproductive health and fertility
    c) To treat infections
    d) To increase muscle mass
34. Which type of stem cells are commonly used in veterinary reproductive treatments?
    a) Embryonic stem cells b) Adult stem cells
    c) Induced pluripotent stem cells d) Cancer stem cells
35. What is the main advantage of using adult stem cells in veterinary gynecology over embryonic stem cells?
    a) Easier to obtain b) Higher differentiation potential
    c) No ethical concerns d) Faster growth
36. In which reproductive condition have stem cell therapies shown potential benefit in veterinary medicine?
    a) Ovarian cysts b) Uterine tumors
    c) Endometritis d) Both a and c
37. What are the potential mechanisms by which MSCs improve fertility in canine sperm?
    a) Increasing sperm size
    b) Secreting proteins like annexin dysferlin, and fibronectin
    c) Reducing sperm count
    d) Altering sperm DNA

38. What is one method used to administer stem cells for treating reproductive issues in animals?
    a) Oral ingestion
    b) Intravenous injection
    c) Direct injection into the reproductive organ
    d) Topical application
39. What is the advantage of using autologous stem cells in veterinary treatments?
    a) Higher differentiation potential
    b) Reduced risk of immune rejection
    c) Easier to harvest
    d) Longer lifespan
40. Stem cell therapy in veterinary gynecology is most advanced in which animal species?
    a) Dogs
    b) Cattle
    c) Horses
    d) Cats
41. In horses, which stem cell source is often used for regenerative reproductive treatments?
    a) Placental tissue
    b) Bone marrow
    c) Hair follicles
    d) Muscle tissue
42. What is the source of embryonic stem cells?
    a) Adult tissues
    b) Bone marrow
    c) Inner cell mass of a blastocyst
    d) Umbilical cord blood
43. What role do stem cells play in treating ovarian cysts in cows?
    a) They replace damaged ovarian tissue
    b) They increase ovarian hormone production
    c) They destroy cystic tissue
    d) They suppress cyst growth
44. In treating endometrial injuries, what type of stem cells are often used?
    a) Mesenchymal stem cells
    b) Hematopoietic stem cells
    c) Neural stem cells
    d) Epithelial stem cells
45. What does the term "niche" refer to in stem cell biology?
    a) The genetic makeup of a stem cell
    b) The microenvironment where stem cells reside
    c) The process of cell differentiation
    d) The type of cell a stem cell will become
46. Which of the following is a challenge in stem cell therapy for animals?
    a) High success rate
    b) Immune rejection
    c) Easy availability of stem cells
    d) Simple differentiation process
47. In which reproductive issue might stem cells be used to help repair damaged uterine lining?
    a) Ovarian tumors
    b) Endometrial atrophy
    c) Cervical stenosis
    d) Testicular degeneration

48. Which of the following is NOT a potential benefit of stem cell therapy in veterinary gynecology?
    a) Improved fertility
    b) Enhanced tissue regeneration
    c) Cure for genetic disorders
    d) Reduction in inflammation
49. What does the term "cell reprogramming" refer to in stem cell biology?
    a) Turning somatic cells into pluripotent stem cells
    b) Enhancing stem cell proliferation
    c) Inducing stem cell apoptosis
    d) Differentiating stem cells into a single type
50. Stem cell banks for animals are primarily used for what purpose?
    a) Research only
    b) Banking financial assets
    c) Storing stem cells for future therapeutic use
    d) Increasing stem cell production in the body
51. What is the typical method used to confirm the success of stem cell therapy in reproductive treatments?
    a) Blood tests
    b) Imaging studies (ultrasound, MRI)
    c) Histopathological examination
    d) All of the above
52. Which reproductive condition in dogs has been experimentally treated using stem cell therapy?
    a) Pyometra
    b) Uterine prolapse
    c) Ovarian neoplasia
    d) Both a and b
53. How are stem cells typically preserved before use in veterinary procedures?
    a) Freeze-drying
    b) Cryopreservation
    c) Chemical preservation
    d) Dehydration
54. What is the primary source of stem cells for autologous therapy in animals?
    a) Donor animals
    b) Embryos
    c) The patient's own tissues
    d) Fetal tissues
55. What is a common method for monitoring the effects of stem cell therapy in animals?
    a) Clinical observation
    b) Histological analysis
    c) Radiographic imaging
    d) All of the above
56. Stem cells are—
    a) Cells that grow uncontrollably
    b) Undifferentiated cells that can turn into other types of cells
    c) The first cell of new living organism (fertilized egg)
    d) Specialized cells that do one job

57. Which of the following statements is true about the stem cells?
   a) Stem cells are specialized type of cells
   b) Stem cells are an undifferentiated form of cells
   c) Stem cells divide and can form different type of differentiated cells which performs different functions
   d) All of these

58. Stem cells can be obtained from___________.
   a) Embryo b) Somatic adult tissue
   c) Umbilical cord blood d) All of the above

59. Which of the following are not source of stem cells?
   a) Umbilical cord blood b) Early embryo
   c) Sperm and eggs d) Certain adult tissue

60. What distinguishes stem cells from other cells?
   a) They are smaller in size
   b) They are specialized for specific function
   c) They are unspecialized
   d) They have a shorter lifespan

61. Which term is used to describe the ability of stem cells to produce more stem cells identical to themselves?
   a) Specialized b) Potency
   c) Differentiation d) Self renewal

62. Which is something that stem cells can repair/cure ?
   a) Sport injuries
   b) Certain disease like Parkinson's disease, multiple sclerosis and diabetes
   c) Bone marrow in cancer patient
   d) All of the above

63. What does "multipotent" mean?
   a) Able to divide and make one kind of cells
   b) Able to divide and make all type of cells
   c) Able to divide and make multiple (but not all) type of cells
   d) Can not divide

64. What is true regarding induced pluripotent stem cells?
   a) They can be turned/forced into other type of cells in lab
   b) They can't be turned into other type of cells
   c) They can be turned back into their original type of cells
   d) All of the above

65. Adult stem can also be referred to as___________.
   a) Somatic stem cells b) Embryonic stem cells
   c) Starter cells d) IPS cells

66. Cells that are able to develop into any type of cell found in the body are referred as_______?
   a) Totipotent b) Plant cell
   c) Pluripotent d) Embryonic cells

67. Embryonic stem cells can differentiate into what kind of cells-
   a) Only cells of brain
   b) All type of specialized cells in the body
   c) Only specialized blood cells
   d) Only cells derived from tissue

68. iPS stem cells are derived from_________________.
   a) Embryonic stem cells b) Adult somatic cells
   c) IVF embryos d) Blastocysts

69. iPS cells are considered as _______________.
   a) Multipotent b) Pluripotent
   c) Totipotent d) Unipotent

70. Which of the following types of stem cells can be made as patient specific stem cells?
   a) Cord-blood stem cells b) iPS cells
   c) SCNT- derived stem cells d) All of the above

71. Blastocysts derived from SCNT could potentially be used for _______________.
   a) Cloning of pets
   b) Patient-specific stem cell therapy
   c) Examining how normal cells can become diseased cells
   d) All of the above

72. Stem cells isolated from later stages in development tend to have____________.
   a) A greater tendency to form tumour
   b) An increased tendency to transdifferentiate
   c) A decrease in potency
   d) An increased ability to survive outside the body

73. Hematopoietic stem cells found in human bone marrow would be classified as_________.
   a) Omnipotent b) Totipotent
   c) Multipotent d) Pluripotent

74. Human ESP are primarily derived from __________________.
   a) Fetal tissue b) Primordial germ cells
   c) Inner cell mass of blastocysts d) 8- cell stage embryo

75. Which refers to the varying ability of stem cells to differentiate into specialized cell types?
   a) Cell potency b) Cell viability
   c) Cell therapy d) Cell regeneration

76. Which of the following is not true about multipotent stem cells?
   a) They can differentiate into any type of cell
   b) They are found in different locations in human body
   c) They are harder to harvest
   d) They are harder to grow in culture

77. Which of the following is not an advantage of iPS cells?
   a) There is no chance of tumour development
   b) They provide patient-specific stem cells
   c) There is no production or destruction of blastocysts
   d) They are considered pluripotent

78. What does pluripotent mean with respect to stem cells?
   a) The same thing as progenitor
   b) They only give rise to red blood cells
   c) They stay the same cell for the rest of their life
   d) They have the potential to become more than one kind of cell

79. The main application of adult stem cells are –
   a) Repairs and replace the damaged tissues
   b) Used for testing various drug
   c) Used in bone marrow transplants to treat specific type of cancers
   d) All of the above

80. Neutral stem cells from the brain can differentiate into which type of cell –
   a) Only specialized brain cells
   b) Specialized brain cells and specialized skin cells
   c) All types of specialized cells
   d) Only specialized blood cells

81. Which best explains why muscle cells are different from blood cells?
   a) Muscle cells are produced by the brain, but blood cells are produced by the heart
   b) Different genes are activated in muscle cells than in blood cells.
   c) Muscles cells experience different environmental influences than blood cells.
   d) A mutation occurs during the development of muscle cells but not in blood cells.

82. Which of the following terms describes a "hollow ball" of about 150 cells which have not yet decided what they will be?
   a) Oocyte b) Zygote
   c) Blastocyst d) Somatic

83. What process best explains how muscle cells and nerve cells can develop from the same fertilized egg?
   a) Genetic engineering b) Survival of the fittest
   c) Differentiation d) Selective breeding

84. A blastocyst has a _______________ which will become placenta and an ______________________ which will become the rest of the embryo.

a) Inner cell mass ; trophoblast
b) Trophoblast; artificial twinning
c) Trophoblast; inner cell mass
d) Somatic cell; enucleated oocyte

85. Which of the following is TRUE about reproductive and therapeutic cloning?

a) Reproductive involves SCNT whereas therapeutic involves artificial twinning
b) Neither involves destroying a blastocyst
c) Both involve SCNT up to the blastocyst stage
d) Reproductive cloning produces embryonic stem cells while therapeutic cloning produces adult stem cells.

86. A specialised group cells which can give rise to one type of cells is termed as ____________.

a) Unipotent
b) Oligopotent
c) Multipotent
d) Totipotent

87. According to International Society for Cellular Therapy, what should be the criteria for cells for use in cellular therapy?

a) Adherence to plastic
b) CD marker expression: Positive CD 73, 90, 105 & Negative CD14, 34, 45, HLA-DR
c) *In vitro* differentiation: Osteoblast, chondroblasts and adipocytes
a) All of the above

88. Which of the following are properties of mesenchymal stem cells?

a) Secretion of neurotrophic and angiogenic factors
b) Increase secretion of trophic factors
c) Growth and differentiation of local stem and progenitor cells
d) All of the above

89. Mesenchymal stem cells were first reported by _________________.

a) Friedenstein and co-workers 1976
b) Chen and co-workers 1960
c) Chena and co-workers 1990
d) Blanc and co-workers 1985

90. Which if the following methods are used for characterisation of stem cells?

a) Magnetic activated cell sorting
b) Fluorescent activated cell sorting
c) Molecular characterisation involving CD markers
d) All of the above

91. What is trilineage differentiation used for mesenchymal stem cells characterisation?

a) Differentiation of stem cells to Osteoblast
b) Differentiation of stem cells to chondroblasts
c) Differentiation of stem cells to adipocytes
d) All of the above

92. What are some of the routes used for cellular therapy for delivery of stem cells?
    a) Intraarterial
    b) Intraperitoneal
    c) Local administration
    d) All of the above
93. Which of the following item is a base medium for culture of stem cells?
    a) FBS
    b) DMEM
    c) Glucose
    d) Non-essential amino acids
94. Which of the following is an example of Unipotent stem cells?
    a) Germ line stem cells
    b) Mesenchymal stem cells
    c) Hematopoietic stem cells
    d) Neural stem cells
95. Which of the following is an example of multipotent stem cells?
    a) Germ line stem cells
    b) Embryonic stem cells
    c) Hematopoietic stem cells
    d) Epidermal stem cells
96. Which of the following is an example of oligopotent stem cells?
    a) Germ line stem cells
    b) Myeloid stem cells
    c) Hematopoietic stem cells
    d) Epidermal stem cells
97. Which of the following is an example of totipotent stem cells?
    a) Zygote
    b) Myeloid stem cells
    c) Hematopoietic stem cells
    d) Epidermal stem cells
98. The zygote remains totipotent until which cell stage?
    a) 16
    b) 32
    c) 64
    d) Till 60 days of gestation
99. Which of the following is an example of pluripotent stem cells?
    a) Zygote
    b) Myeloid stem cells
    c) Hematopoietic stem cells
    d) Embryonic stem cells
100. Spores are coming under what type of stem cells?
    a) Totipotent stem cells
    b) Pluripotent stem cells
    c) Oligopotent stem cells
    d) Unipotent

References

Barry, F. P. and Murphy, J. M. 2004. 2004. Mesenchymal stem cells: clinical applications and biological characterization. Int. J. Biochem. Cell Biol. 36: 568–584.

Blanc, K.L. and Davies, L. c. 2018. MSCs—cells with many sides. Cytotherapy. 20: 273–278.

Kim, E.J., Kim, N. and Cho, S.G.2013. The potential use of mesenchymal stem cells in hematopoietic stem cell transplantation. Expl. Mol. Med. 45:e2.

Friedenstein, a.J., Gorskaja, U..F and Julagina, N.N. 1976. Fibroblast precursors in normal and irradiated mouse hematopoietic organs. Exp. Hematol. 4: 267–274.

Remya, V., Kumar, N., Ninu, a.R., Radhika, S., Kutty, M.V.H. and Maiti, S.K. 2014. Isolation and culture of bone marrow derived mesenchymal cells from goat. In d. J. Sci. Res. Tech. 2(3): 60-62.

Answer Key

1	a	2	a	3	c	4	b	5	d	6	c	7	c
8	d	9	b	10	b	11	b	12	c	13	b	14	c
15	c	16	c	17	d	18	b	19	b	20	d	21	a
22	b	23	b	24	b	25	a	26	a	27	b	28	a
29	b	30	b	31	c	32	c	33	b	34	b	35	c
36	d	37	b	38	c	39	b	40	c	41	b	42	c
43	a	44	a	45	b	46	b	47	b	48	c	49	a
50	c	51	d	52	d	53	b	54	c	55	d	56	b
57	d	58	d	59	c	60	c	61	d	62	d	63	c
64	a	65	a	66	a	67	b	68	b	69	b	70	d
71	d	72	c	73	c	74	c	75	a	76	a	77	c
78	d	79	d	80	a	81	b	82	c	83	c	84	c
85	c	86	a	87	b	88	d	89	a	90	d	91	d
92	d	93	b	94	a	95	c	96	b	97	a	98	a
99	d	100	a										

10

Basic Body Plan Development

Jasvinder Singh Sasan, Shalini Suri and Kamal Sarma

Division of Veterinary Anatomy, Faculty of Veterinary Sciences and Animal Husbandry, Sher-e-Kashmir University of Agricultural Sciences and Technology of Jammu, Jammu and Kashmir

---

The formation of the mammalian body plan is regulated by highly conserved gene regulatory networks. During this developmental stage, the notochord and primitive node play critical roles in establishing the cranial-caudal axis and left-right asymmetry. Ectoderm, the outer germ layer, differentiates into neuroectoderm and surface ectoderm. Neuroectodermal cells move from the developing neural tube's lateral edges to a dorsolateral position. These neuroectodermal cells are known as neural crest cells. The central nervous system originates from the neural tube, whereas the peripheral nervous system originates from both the neural tube and the neural crest. Mesoderm cells proliferate and develops into three separate components: the paraxial, intermediate, and lateral plate of mesoderm. The paraxial mesoderm cells form whorl-like aggregations known as somitomeres on both sides of the neural plate. Paraxial mesoderm organises into separate blocks known as somites caudal to the seventh somitomere. Somatic cells make up the vast majority of the axial skeleton, accompanying muscle, and covering dermis. The embryonic gut tube, developing respiratory system, and accompanying glands all develop from endoderm, the inner germ layer. Endoderm is also responsible for the epithelial linings of the urinary bladder, middle ear, and auditory tube. Endoderm also gives rise to the parenchymal cells of the thyroid, parathyroid glands, pancreas, and liver.

Multiple Choice Questions

1. At the end of gastrulation, developing embryo is:
   a) Elongated b) Pear shaped
   c) Oval d) Cylindrical
2. Notochord is longitudinal column of:
   a) Ectoderm b) Mesoderm
   c) Endoderm d) All of the above
3. Notochord arises from:
   a) Primitive groove b) Primitive ridge
   c) Primitive node d) None of the above
4. Notochord establishes which axis of developing embryo:
   a) Cranio-caudal b) Latero-medial
   c) Dorso-ventral d) None of the above

5. Which of the following above notochord proliferates to form neural plate:
   a) Par-axial mesoderm
   b) Endoderm
   c) Ectoderm
   d) Intermediate mesoderm
6. Central nervous system develops from:
   a) Neural tube
   b) Neural crest
   c) Both a & b
   d) None of the above
7. Peripheral nervous system develops from:
   a) Neural tube
   b) Neural crest
   c) Both a & b
   d) None of the above
8. Neural crest cells are located:
   a) Dorso-medial to neural tube
   b) Ventro-medial to neural tube
   c) Ventro-lateral to neural tube
   d) Dorso-lateral to neural tube
9. Otic placodes give rise to:
   a) Nasal chamber
   b) Lens
   c) Inner ear
   d) External ear
10. Under the influence of neural tube and neural crest, surface ectodermal cells in cephalic region form thickenings known as:
   a) Vesicle
   b) Placode
   c) Somite
   d) Somitomere
11. Somitomere develops from:
   a) Neural crest cells
   b) Paraxial mesoderm
   c) Intermediate mesoderm
   d) Neural tube
12. Epithelial lining of primitive gut develops from:
   a) Ectoderm
   b) Par-axial mesoderm
   c) Intermediate mesoderm
   d) Endoderm
13. Epithelial lining of urinary bladder and middle ear develops from:
   a) Ectoderm
   b) Par-axial mesoderm
   c) Intermediate mesoderm
   d) Endoderm
14. Which of the following develops from endoderm:
   a) Parenchymal cells of liver
   b) Epithelial lining of auditory tube
   c) Parathyroid glands
   d) All of the above
15. Which of the following statement is incorrect:
   a) Ectoderm directly above notochord gives rise to neural plate
   b) Mesoderm lies between epiblast and hypoblast
   c) Neural plate forms neural groove
   d) Following formation of neural tube, superficial cell layers is known as neuro-ectoderm
16. Development of somitomere begins in:
   a) Caudal region
   b) Cephalic region
   c) Mid-thoracic region
   d) Lumbar region

17. Paraxial, intermediate and lateral plate are part of:
    a) Notochord b) Mesoderm
    c) Neuro-ectoderm d) Endoderm
18. Which of the following lines the embryonic gut tube and the developing respiratory tract:
    a) Notochord b) Mesoderm
    c) Neuro-ectoderm d) Endoderm
19. On either side of the neural plate, cells of the paraxial mesoderm form whorl-like aggregations called:
    a) Somite b) Somitomere
    c) Placode d) Neural crest cells
20. Sclerotome, dermatome and myotome are part of:
    a) Placode b) Somites
    c) Neural crest cells d) Neural tube
21. Caudal to the which somitomere, paraxial mesoderm becomes organized into somites:
    a) 3rd b) 7th
    c) 9th d) 13th
22. Number of occipital somites in canine embryo:
    a) Four b) Eight
    c) Ten d) Seven
23. Number of cervical somites in canine embryo:
    a) Four b) Eight
    c) Ten d) Seven
24. Number of thoracic somites in canine embryo:
    a) Thirteen b) Eight
    c) Ten d) Seven
25. Number of lumbar somites in canine embryo:
    a) Four b) Eight
    c) Ten d) Seven
26. Number of sacral somites in canine embryo:
    a) Three b) Eight
    c) Ten d) Seven
27. Mesoderm lateral to the somites forms a column of cells is known as:
    a) Par-axial mesoderm b) Intermediate mesoderm
    c) Chorda-mesoderm d) Notochord
28. Somatic layer and splanchnic layer are part of:
    a) Par-axial mesoderm b) Intermediate mesoderm
    c) Lateral plate of mesoderm d) Notochord

29. Somatopleure is formed by fusion of:
    a) Somatic layer and ectoderm
    b) Somatic layer and endoderm
    c) Splanchnic layer and ectoderm
    d) Splanchnic layer and endoderm
30. Splanchnopleure is formed by fusion of:
    a) Somatic layer and ectoderm
    b) Somatic layer and endoderm
    c) Splanchnic layer and ectoderm
    d) Splanchnic layer and endoderm
31. Which is true regarding pharyngeal arches:
    a) Develops in cranio-caudal direction
    b) Develops in caudo-cranial direction
    c) Develops between the foregut and surface ectoderm
    d) Both a & c
32. Appearance of primitive streak occurs at which part of future embryo proper:
    a) Cranial pole
    b) Caudal pole
    c) Any part of embryo
    d) None of the above
33. Trophectoderm and the extra-embryonic somatic mesoderm form:
    a) Chorion
    b) Amnion
    c) Allantois
    d) Yolk sac
34. Parietal portions of the peritoneum and pleura develops from:
    a) Somatic mesoderm
    b) Splanchnic mesoderm
    c) Endoderm
    d) Notochord
35. Visceral portions of the peritoneum and pleura develops from:
    a) Somatic mesoderm
    b) Splanchnic mesoderm
    c) Endoderm
    d) Notochord
36. Which of the following is true regarding notochord:
    a) Establishes the anterior-posterior embryonic axis
    b) Formed by epiblast cells ingressing through the primitive node
    c) Located at the anterior end of the primitive streak
    d) All of the above
37. Mesodermal structure located just anterior to the tip of the notochord is:
    a) Somite
    b) Placode
    c) Somitomere
    d) Prechordal plate
38. In large animal species, on average, somites are formed at a rate of:
    a) About six pairs a day
    b) About one pair a day
    c) About ten pairs a day
    d) About thirteen pairs a day
39. Ventro-medial part of the somite is:
    a) Dermatome
    b) Myotome
    c) Nephrotome
    d) Sclerotome

40. Dorso-lateral part of each somite is:
    a) Sclerotome
    b) Dermamyotome
    c) Nephrotome
    d) Both a & c
41. Which part of somite is associated with vertebral column formation:
    a) Dermatome
    b) Myotome
    c) Nephrotome
    d) Sclerotome
42. Which part of somite is associated with dermal and muscle tissue formation:
    a) Sclerotome
    b) Dermamyotome
    c) Nephrotome
    d) Both a & c
43. Intermediate mesoderm in the cervical and cranial thoracic regions forms segmental cell clusters known as:
    a) Somitomere
    b) Somite
    c) Nephrotomere
    d) Nephrogenic cord
44. Remnant of notochord in adult is:
    a) Annulus fibrosus of intervertebral disc
    b) Nucleus pulposus of intervertebral disc
    c) Ligamentum nuchae
    d) Ligamentum flava
45. Rathke's pouch is associated with development of:
    a) Pineal gland
    b) Pituitary gland
    c) Adrenal gland
    d) Thyroid gland

Answer Key

1	b	2	b	3	c	4	a	5	c	6	a	7	c
8	d	9	c	10	b	11	b	12	d	13	d	14	d
15	d	16	b	17	b	18	d	19	b	20	b	21	b
22	a	23	b	24	a	25	d	26	a	27	b	28	c
29	a	30	d	31	d	32	b	33	a	34	a	35	b
36	d	37	d	38	a	39	d	40	b	41	d	42	b
43	c	44	b	45	b								

11

Coelomic Cavities Development

Archana Mahapatra[1], Sakshi[2] and Tanmoy Rana[3]

[1]*Department of Veterinary Anatomy, Faculty of Veterinary and Animal Sciences Institute of Agricultural Sciences, Rajiv Gandhi South Campus, Banaras Hindu University RGSC, BHU, Barkachha, India*

[2]*Division of Medicine, ICAR- IVRI, Bareilly, India*

[3]*Department of Veterinary Clinical Complex, West Bengal University of Animal and Fishery Sciences, Kolkata, India*

Introduction

At the end of gastrulation, the mesoderm of the developing embryo differentiates into three regions: paraxial, intermediate, and lateral mesoderm. These regions play crucial roles in the formation of various body structures. As development proceeds, clefts form in the lateral mesoderm, which later coalesce to form a cavity. This cavity splits the lateral mesoderm into two layers: the somatic (outer) layer and the splanchnic (inner) layer. The space between these layers on each side of the midline becomes known as the coelomic cavity. These left and right coelomic cavities extend cranially, meet in front of the developing neural and cardiogenic plates, and fuse to form a horseshoe-shaped coelomic cavity.

The walls of the developing coelomic cavity have two layers. The outer layer consists of somatic mesoderm, which fuses with ectoderm to form the somatopleure. The inner layer consists of splanchnic mesoderm, which fuses with endoderm to form the splanchnopleure. The mesodermal cells lining the coelomic cavity differentiate into a simple squamous epithelium called mesothelium. As cranial, caudal, and lateral folding occurs during embryonic development, the convex region of the horseshoe-shaped coelom eventually takes a ventral position to the foregut and developing heart, forming the primordium of the pericardial cavity.

The developing coelomic cavities, initially continuous with one another at the umbilicus, become separated into intra-embryonic and extra-embryonic regions. The intra-embryonic coelom gives rise to the pericardial, pleural, and peritoneal cavities, while the extra-embryonic coelom is associated with the developing fetal membranes. As the embryo folds laterally, the coelomic cavity divides into two separate components.

The pleural cavities, which surround the developing lungs, are initially part of the pleuro-pericardial cavity, alongside the developing heart. As mesodermal folds, known as pleuro-pericardial folds, grow medially, they enclose the common cardinal veins and the phrenic nerves. These folds eventually separate the pleuro-pericardial cavity into two parts: the pleural cavities dorsally, and the pericardial cavities ventrally. The developing lungs grow into the pleural cavities, and as they expand, the mesothelium forms the visceral pleura (lining the lungs) and the parietal pleura (lining the wall of the pleural cavity).

The pericardial cavity, where the heart develops, is initially suspended by a dorsal mesocardium (a fold of mesothelium) and anchored by a ventral mesocardium. The ventral mesocardium degenerates early in development, and as a result, the dorsal mesocardium also atrophies. This leads to the formation of a single pericardial cavity. At this stage, the heart is suspended solely by the blood vessels entering and leaving the heart. The pericardial sac consists of two layers: the visceral layer, which surrounds the heart, and the parietal layer, which lines the thoracic wall. The outer layer of the pericardium is formed by a fibrous layer that fuses with structures such as the diaphragm or sternum (depending on the species), and the phrenic nerves are enclosed within this fibrous structure.

The diaphragm plays a crucial role in separating the thoracic and abdominal cavities. During early development, the pleuro-pericardial cavity communicates with the embryonic coelom. As cranio-caudal folding progresses, a mesodermal aggregation called the septum transversum moves from a cranial position (above the developing heart) to a caudal position, forming a transverse partition called the diaphragm. This partition separates the pleuro-pericardial cavity from the peritoneal cavity. The pleuro-peritoneal folds develop from the lateral body wall and grow medially to fuse with the mesoesophagus and the septum transversum. This fusion leads to the formation of the primordial diaphragm, which later develops into the muscular diaphragm. The diaphragm is innervated by the phrenic nerve, originating from cervical spinal nerves, while the muscular rim of the diaphragm is innervated by thoracic and lumbar spinal nerves.

Congenital anomalies of the diaphragm can occur when the components do not fuse properly, resulting in a persistent opening between the abdominal and thoracic cavities. This can lead to congenital diaphragmatic hernias, where abdominal organs may enter the thoracic cavity. Two main types of congenital hernias are recognized: pleuro-peritoneal herniation and peritoneal-pericardial herniation. Pleuro-peritoneal herniation occurs due to the failure of the pleuro-peritoneal folds to develop or fuse properly, allowing communication between the abdominal and thoracic cavities, usually on the left side. Peritoneal-pericardial herniation, more common in domestic animals, is associated with a defect in the septum transversum, which results in abnormal communication between the peritoneal and pericardial cavities.

In the developing abdominal cavity, the gut is initially suspended by both dorsal and ventral mesenteries. These mesenteries connect the developing intestine to the abdominal wall. As the gut develops, the ventral mesentery atrophies in certain regions, while the dorsal mesentery persists. This allows the gut to grow and undergo partial rotation. As the mesenteries evolve, they become structures known as ligaments, which connect organs to each other or to the body wall. The peritoneum, a mesothelial membrane that lines the abdominal cavity, forms these mesenteries and ligaments. The peritoneal cavity, which contains a small amount of peritoneal fluid, is the space between the parietal and visceral layers of the peritoneum.

The concept of omenta refers to peritoneal folds that connect the stomach to surrounding structures. The dorsal and ventral mesogastrium suspend the stomach and are altered by the stomach's rotation during development. As the stomach rotates to the left, the dorsal mesogastrium elongates and forms the greater omentum, which consists of two peritoneal folds enclosing a cavity known as the omental bursa. The omental bursa communicates with the peritoneal cavity via the epiploic foramen. The spleen develops from mesodermal aggregations in the superficial leaf of the greater omentum, and the greater omentum forms the gastrosplenic ligament (connecting the spleen to the stomach) and the renosplenic ligament (connecting the spleen to the kidney).

The pancreas also develops within the omentum, specifically in the superficial fold of the greater omentum. The liver grows into the ventral mesogastrium, dividing it into two parts. These folds form the lesser omentum, which connects the stomach to the liver, and the falciform ligament, which connects the liver to the ventral body wall.

In summary, the embryonic development of the mesoderm, coelomic cavities, and associated structures is a complex process that results in the formation of key body systems. The mesodermal layers give rise to the pericardial, pleural, and peritoneal cavities, as well as vital structures like the diaphragm and omenta. This process is crucial for the correct development of the thoracic and abdominal cavities, ensuring proper organ positioning and function. Congenital anomalies in these processes, such as diaphragmatic hernias, can lead to significant developmental issues.

Multiple Choice Questions

1. Differentiation of the ________________leads to formation of a cavity (coelom) between the two layers of lateral plate mesoderm.
   a) Ectoderm b) Mesoderm
   c) Endoderm d) Primitive streak
2. ________________________ develops into pericardial, pleural and peritoneal cavities.
   a) Intraembryonic coelom b) Extraembryonic coelom
   c) Notochord d) Nucleus pulposus
3. ________________partly separates the developing thoracic and abdominal cavities, which communicate with each other via the pleuro-peritoneal canals.
   a) Septum primum b) Septum secundum
   c) Septum transversum d) Septum trabeculae
4. In mammals, development of ________________ leads to complete separation of the thoracic and abdominal cavities.
   a) Diaphragm b) Liver
   c) Lumbar vertebra d) Somite
5. The lateral walls of the intra embryonic coelomic cavity are composed of
   a) Somatic mesoderm
   b) Somatic mesoderm and endoderm
   c) Splanchnic mesoderm and ectoderm
   d) Splanchnic mesoderm and endoderm
6. The medial walls of the intra embryonic coelomic cavity are composed of
   a) Somatic mesoderm and ectoderm
   b) Somatic mesoderm and endoderm

c) Splanchnic mesoderm and ectoderm
d) Splanchnic mesoderm

7. The lateral wall of the coelomic cavity are composed of somatic mesoderm which fuses with ectoderm and forms
   a) Somatopleuare
   b) Splanchopleuare
   c) Pleura
   d) Pericardium
8. The medial wall of the coelomic cavity are composed of splanchnic mesoderm which fuses with endoderm and forms
   a) Somatopleuare
   b) Splanchnopleuare
   c) Pleura
   d) Pericardium
9. The mesodermal cells lining the coelomic cavity differentiate into a simple squamous epithelium referred to as
   a) Mesothelium
   b) Endothelium
   c) Mesosalpinx
   d) Endometrium
10. Which of the following statement(s) is/ are incorrect
    a) Following cranial caudal and lateral folding of the embryo, the convex region of the horseshoe-shaped coelom occupies a position ventral to the foregut and the developing heart, and gives rise to the primordium of the pericardial cavity.
    b) The right and left limbs of the coelomic cavity are connected to the pericardial cavity by the pericardial–peritoneal canals
    c) The intra-embryonic coelom gives rise to the pericardial,pleural and peritoneal cavities.
    d) The intra-embryonic coelom is associated with the developing foetal membranes
11. The intraembryonic and extra-embryonic coelomic cavities, are initially continuous at the
    a) Umbilicus
    b) Urachus
    c) Amnion
    d) Chorion
12. _______________ gives rise to the parietal portions of the peritoneum and pleura
    a) Somatic mesoderm
    b) Visceral mesoderm
    c) Endoderm
    d) Ectoderm
13. Together, the trophectoderm and the extra-embryonic somatic mesoderm will form the outer layers of the embryonic part of the placenta i.e.
    a) Amnion
    b) Chorion
    c) Annantois
    d) Yolk sac
14. The cavity formed between the somatic and visceral mesoderm is referred to as the
    a) Amnion
    b) Chorion
    c) Coelom
    d) Yolksac
15. Coelomic cavity is
    a) Mesoderm in nature
    b) Ectoderm in nature
    c) Endoderm in nature
    d) Meso-ectoderm in nature

16. The cavities between the two layers of mesoderm on the left and right sides are referred to as __________
    a) Gastric cavity b) Coelomic cavity
    c) Mesodermal cavity d) All of the above
17. The shape of coelomic cavity is
    a) A horseshoe-shaped b) Amoeboid shaped
    c) Boat shaped d) Funnel shaped
18. The _____ walls of the coelomic cavity are composed of somatic mesoderm which fuses with ectoderm, forming somatopleure
    a) Dorsal walls b) Ventral walls
    c) Lateral walls d) Paraventral walls
19. The medial walls of coelomic cavity are composed of ______ which fuses with endoderm, forming splanchnopleure
    a) Splanchnic ectoderm b) Splanchnic endoderm
    c) Somatic mesoderm d) Splanchnic mesoderm
20. The tissue lining the coelomic cavity is called
    a) Endothelium b) Mesothelium
    c) Endocolium d) Mesocoelium
21. The mesothelium is _________ tissue in nature
    a) Simple stratified epithelium b) Simple columnar epithelium
    c) Simple squamous epithelium d) Stratified stratified epithelium
22. The right and left limbs of the coelomic cavity are connected to the ____ cavity by the pericardial–peritoneal canals
    a) Peritoneal cavity b) Pleural cavity
    c) Pericardial cavity d) All the above cavity
23. The extra-embryonic coelom is associated with the developing ______
    a) Abdominal organs b) Thoracic organs
    c) Foetal membranes d) Abdominal viscera
24. In dogs and cats, a fibrous layer anchors the pericardium to the developing ______ is known as ________
    a) Diaphragm, sterno-pericardial ligament
    b) Sternum, sterno-pericardial ligament
    c) Diaphragm, phrenico-pericardial ligament
    d) Sternum, phrenico-pericardial ligament
25. In horse and cattle, a fibrous layer anchors the pericardium to the developing ______ is known as ________
    a) Diaphragm, sterno-pericardial ligament
    b) Sternum, sterno-pericardial ligament
    c) Diaphragm, phrenico-pericardial ligament
    d) Sternum, phrenico-pericardial ligament

26. The mesothelium in direct contact with the developing lungs is referred to as _____ pleura while the mesothelium in contact with the wall of the pleural cavity is called the _____ pleura

a) Pleural, pleural
b) Visceral, pleural
c) Pleural, Visceral
d) Visceral, Visceral

27. The heart is initially suspended by ______ dorsal fold of mesothelium, the dorsal mesocardium

a) Single
b) Double
c) Triple
d) Quadruple

28. All the structures within the thoracic cavity are contained within the mediastinal space except

a) Lungs
b) Caudal vena cava
c) Right phrenic nerve
d) All of the above

29. The partition formed by fusion of the pleuroperitoneal folds, the dorsal mesothelial fold suspending the oesophagus and the septum transversum, constitutes the ________

a) Diaphragm
b) Sternum
c) Mediastinum
d) Falciform ligament

30. The musculature of the central region of the diaphragm is innervated by ventral branches of ________ nerves which form the left and right phrenic nerves

a) Cranial cervical nerve
b) Caudal cervical nerve
c) Cranial carotid nerve
d) Caudal carotid nerve

31. Aortic hiatus is opening for passage of

a) Aorta
b) Azygous vein
c) Thoracic duct
d) All of the above

32. Oesophageal hiatus is passage for

a) Esophagus
b) Dorsal branches of vagus nerve
c) Ventral branches of vagus nerve
d) All of the above

33. Caval foramen is opening for

a) Cranialvena cava
b) Aorta
c) Thoracic duct
d) Caudal vena cava

34. Congenital diaphragmatic herniation is

a) When abdominal viscera pass through this opening into the thoracic cavity
b) There can be pleuro-peritoneal herniation
c) There can be peritoneal–pericardial herniation
d) All of the above

35. Which type of congenital diaphragmatic herniation is common in dog and cats

a) Pleuro-peritoneal herniation
b) Peritoneal–pericardial herniation
c) Both of above
d) None of the above

36. The most common form of diaphragmatic herniation observed in small animal veterinary practice usually results from

a) Pathological causes b) Traumatic causes
c) Nutritional causes d) Congenital causes

37. In the developing abdominal cavity, the gut is suspended by folds of _______ between the left and right coelomic cavities

a) Splanchnic ectoderm b) Splanchnic endoderm
c) Splanchnic mesoderm d) None of the above

38. The mesothelium which lines the abdominal wall is known as

a) Pericardium b) Peritoneum
c) Omentum d) Mesentery

39. Folds of peritoneum which surround the intestine and connect it to the body wall are referred to as

a) Omentum b) Ligament
c) Mesentery d) Pericardium

40. The folds of peritoneum which attach organs to each other, or attach organs to the body wall, are referred to as

a) Mesentery b) Ligament
c) Omentum d) Pericardium

41. If the organs are enclosed by the fold of peritoneum then the organs are classified as

a) Inter peritoneal b) Intra-peritoneal
c) Retroperitoneal d) Retrograde peritoneal

42. Organs which are partly covered by peritoneum are known as

a) Inter- peritoneal b) Intraperitoneal
c) Retroperitoneal d) Retrograde peritoneal

43. The fold of peritoneum that attaches an organ to the stomach

a) Ligament b) Mesentery
c) Omentum d) Mesothelium

44. During rotation of the stomach to the left, the dorsal mesogastrium elongates and form a pouch-like double fold enclosing a cavity known as

a) Ligamental bursa b) Mesentery
c) Omental bursa d) Mesentery bursa

45. The omental bursa communicates with the peritoneal cavity through an opening known as

a) Aortic hiatus b) Esophagus hiatus
c) Epiploic foramen d) Gastric foramen

46. The fold of omentum which attaches the spleen to stomach is known as

a) Gastrosplenic ligament b) Renosplenic ligament
c) Renosplenic mesentery d) Gastrosplenic mesentery

47. The fold of omentum which attaches the spleen to kidney is known as
    a) Gastrosplenic ligamnent b) Renosplenic ligament
    c) Renosplenic mesentery d) Gastrosplenic mesentery
48. __________ folding of the embryo divides the developing embryonic coelom into intra-embryonic and extra- embryonic regions
    a) Dorsal b) Ventral
    c) Lateral d) Mid ventral
49. Which of the statement(s) is/are correct for coelomic cavity
    a) The cavity within bones
    b) A body cavity between the ectoderm and mesoderm
    c) A fluid filled cavity lined by mesothelium
    d) The cavity will in the intestine
50. Most prominently developed coelomic cavity is found in
    a) Protozoa b) Arthropoda
    c) Vertebrates d) Porifera
51. What is the primary function of coelomic cavity
    a) Circulation of blood
    b) Space for internal organs and their movement
    c) Protection of abdominal organs
    d) Energy storage
52. Which of the following structure is part of the coelomic cavity in mammals
    a) Pleural cavity b) Pericardial cavity
    c) Peritoneal cavity d) All of the above
53. In birds, the coelomic cavity is divided into
    a) One compartment b) Two compartments
    c) Three compartments d) Four compartments
54. The function of coelomic fluid is
    a) To provide nutrients to organ b) To act as lubricant
    c) To facilitate the exchange of gases d) All of the above
55. Which embryonic layer is origin of coelomic cavity?
    a) Ectoderm b) Mesoderm
    c) Ectoderm d) Blastoderm
56. Which of the following animals lack a true coelomic cavity?
    a) Earthworm b) Mammals
    c) Flatworms d) Amphibians
57. In mammals, which structure separates the thoracic cavity from abdominal cavity
    a) Pericardium b) Pleura
    c) Diaphragm d) Mesentery

58. The coelomic cavity in birds is divided into

a) Pericardial and pleural cavities
b) Peritoneal cavity and air sacs
c) Both a and b
d) Undivided coelomic cavity

59. Which structure allows the movement of the internal organ in coelomic cavity

a) Omentum
b) Coelomic fluid
c) Mesentery
d) Ligament

60. What is the primary function of the epiblast during early development?

a) To form the extra-embryonic membranes
b) To contribute to the formation of the three somatic germ layers: ectoderm, mesoderm, and endoderm
c) To form the trophoblast and hypoblast
d) To develop into the primitive gut

61. The term 'gastrulation' refers to:

a) The process of forming the amniotic cavity
b) The formation of the primordial germ cells
c) The formation of the primitive gut and germ layers
d) The differentiation of the trophoblast into the extra-embryonic tissues

62. In which species does the mesamnion disappear, leaving no connection between the amnion and chorion?

a) Ruminants
b) Pigs
c) Horses and carnivores
d) Birds

63. What happens to the amnion during parturition in pigs and ruminants?

a) The amnion remains intact until after birth
b) The amnion is removed manually to prevent suffocation
c) The amnion is torn during birth because the mesamnion persists
d) The amnion fuses with the allantois before birth

64. The intra-embryonic mesoderm arises from:

a) Cells that ingressed through the primitive streak but remain between the epiblast and hypoblast
b) The primitive gut during gastrulation
c) The trophoblast and extra-embryonic mesoderm
d) The epiblast and hypoblast only

65. What is the coelom, and where is it located initially?

a) A cavity between the somatic and visceral mesoderm, located entirely within the embryonic disc
b) A cavity that forms between the somatic and visceral mesoderm, initially located outside the embryonic disc
c) A membrane surrounding the developing embryo
d) A space between the endoderm and ectoderm that forms the gut

66. The somatic and visceral mesoderm give rise to which of the following?
    a) Somatic mesoderm forms the inner lining of the gastrointestinal tract; visceral mesoderm forms the body wall
    b) Somatic mesoderm forms the outer layers of the placenta; visceral mesoderm forms the body cavities
    c) Somatic mesoderm forms the parietal portions of the peritoneum and pleura; visceral mesoderm forms the visceral portions of these serous membranes
    d) Both somatic and visceral mesoderm contribute equally to the development of the heart

67. The extra-embryonic coelom (exocoelom) is initially located:
    a) Within the embryonic disc
    b) Between the epiblast and hypoblast
    c) Outside the embryonic disc
    d) Between the primitive streak and the mesoderm

68. During the development of the mesoderm, the primitive streak becomes more posteriorly located due to:
    a) The rapid growth of the epiblast
    b) Differential growth of the embryonic disc
    c) The formation of the extra-embryonic mesoderm
    d) The closure of the coelom

69. The trophectoderm and extra-embryonic somatic mesoderm contribute to the formation of:
    a) The developing neural tube
    b) The extra-embryonic coelom
    c) The outer layers of the embryonic part of the placenta, the chorion
    d) The mesodermal layers of the heart

70. During the folding process, the coelom becomes subdivided into which of the following cavities?
    a) Peritoneal, pleural, and pericardial cavities
    b) Amniotic and allantoic cavities
    c) Endodermal and ectodermal cavities
    d) Chorionic and mesodermal cavities

71. The somatopleura contributes to the formation of:
    a) The wall of the primitive gut
    b) The lateral and ventral body wall, with the somatic mesoderm lining the inside
    c) The inner lining of the primitive gut
    d) The amnion and chorion

72. The splanchnopleura forms which part of the embryo?
   a) The lateral and ventral body wall
   b) The wall of the primitive gut and its derivatives
   c) The epidermis of the body
   d) The pericardial cavity and its lining
73. In the formation of the primitive gut, the inner lining is provided by:
   a) The visceral mesoderm
   b) The ectoderm
   c) The endoderm
   d) The somatic mesoderm
74. The serous membranes lining the parietal surfaces of the peritoneal, pleural, and pericardial cavities are derived from:
   a) The splanchnic mesoderm
   b) The visceral mesoderm
   c) The somatic mesoderm
   d) The ectoderm
75. The serous membranes covering the organs in the peritoneal, pleural, and pericardial cavities are derived from:
   a) The ectoderm
   b) The somatic mesoderm
   c) The visceral mesoderm
   d) The endoderm
76. The allantois is formed during which week of development?
   a) First week
   b) Second or third week, depending on the species
   c) Fourth week
   d) Fifth week
77. In ruminants and pigs, the allantois takes on which shape?
   a) Circular
   b) T-shaped
   c) Y-shaped
   d) U-shaped
78. In the T-shaped allantois, where is the top bar of the "T" located?
   a) At the anterior end of the embryo
   b) Just caudal to the embryo proper
   c) Alongside the primitive streak
   d) At the anterior end of the umbilical cord
79. The allantoic duct connects which two structures?
   a) The primitive gut and the yolk sac
   b) The allantoic cavity and the hindgut
   c) The primitive streak and the embryonic disc
   d) The ectoderm and the mesoderm
80. The allantoic duct becomes incorporated into which structure as a result of embryonic foldings?
   a) The placenta
   b) The amniotic cavity
   c) The umbilical cord
   d) The yolk sac

81. At the end of gastrulation, the embryonic mesoderm is divided into which three regions?
   a) Paraxial, intermediate, and lateral mesoderm
   b) Somatic, splanchnic, and intermediate mesoderm
   c) Ectoderm, mesoderm, and endoderm
   d) Somatic, splanchnic, and parietal mesoderm
82. What is the term used for the cavities formed between the two layers of lateral mesoderm?
   a) Coelomic cavities
   b) Pleural cavities
   c) Peritoneal cavities
   d) Pericardial cavities
83. The coelomic cavities on either side of the midline meet and fuse in front of which developing structures?
   a) Primitive gut and lungs
   b) Neural and cardiogenic plates
   c) Amniotic cavity and yolk sac
   d) Ectoderm and mesoderm layers
84. The lateral walls of the coelomic cavity are composed of which type of mesoderm?
   a) Somatic mesoderm
   b) Splanchnic mesoderm
   c) Parietal mesoderm
   d) Intermediate mesoderm
85. The medial walls of the coelomic cavity are composed of which type of mesoderm?
   a) Somatic mesoderm
   b) Splanchnic mesoderm
   c) Parietal mesoderm
   d) Intermediate mesoderm
86. The mesodermal cells lining the coelomic cavity differentiate into what type of epithelium?
   a) Endothelium
   b) Mesothelium
   c) Ectodermal epithelium
   d) Mucosal epithelium
87. The cranial portion of the horseshoe-shaped coelom gives rise to which of the following?
   a) Peritoneal cavity
   b) Pericardial cavity
   c) Pleural cavity
   d) Allantois
88. The pleuro-pericardial folds contain which important structures?
   a) Phrenic nerves and common cardinal veins
   b) Visceral pleura and pericardial cavity
   c) Parietal pleura and developing heart
   d) Developing lungs and mesothelium
89. After the pleuro-pericardial folds meet, they divide the pleuro-pericardial cavity into which two cavities?
   a) Pleural and peritoneal cavities
   b) Pericardial and pleural cavities
   c) Pleural and pericardial cavities, dorsally and ventrally
   d) Visceral and parietal cavities

90. The mesothelium in contact with the developing lungs is referred to as:
    a) Parietal pleura
    b) Visceral pleura
    c) Pericardium
    d) Mesothelium

91. The heart is initially suspended by which structure?
    a) Ventral mesocardium
    b) Dorsal mesocardium
    c) Fibrous pericardium
    d) Both dorsal and ventral mesocardium

92. What happens to the dorsal and ventral mesocardium during heart development?
    a) Both mesocardia persist and anchor the heart
    b) The ventral mesocardium atrophies, followed by the dorsal mesocardium
    c) The dorsal mesocardium forms the fibrous pericardium
    d) Both mesocardia develop into the mediastinum

93. What forms the fibrous layer of the pericardium?
    a) Dorsal mesocardium
    b) Parietal pleura
    c) Fusion of the inner body wall layers and the pleuro-pericardial folds
    d) Septum transversum

94. In dogs and cats, the fibrous pericardium is referred to as the:
    a) Phrenico-pericardial ligament
    b) Sternal ligament
    c) Pleuro-peritoneal canal
    d) Mediastinum

95. What is the name of the mesodermal tissue that forms a partition separating the pleural cavities?
    a) Mediastinum
    b) Septum transversum
    c) Mesoesophagus
    d) Pleuro-peritoneal folds

96. What structure separates the pleuro-pericardial cavity from the developing peritoneal cavity?
    a) Mediastinum
    b) Pleuro-peritoneal folds
    c) Septum transversum
    d) Diaphragm

97. What results from the fusion of the pleuro-peritoneal folds, mesoesophagus, and septum transversum?
    a) The pericardial cavity
    b) The primordial diaphragm
    c) The thoracic cavity
    d) The fibrous pericardium

98. The muscular rim of the diaphragm is derived from which source?
    a) Mesoderm from the pleuro-peritoneal folds
    b) Mesoderm from the developing thoracic cavity
    c) Mesoderm derived from the body wall
    d) Mesoderm from the septum transversum

99. What does the primordial diaphragm partially separate?
    a) The pericardial and pleural cavities
    b) The pericardial cavity from the peritoneal cavity
    c) The pleural and peritoneal cavities
    d) The thoracic and abdominal cavities

100. The pleuro-pericardial folds are associated with which structures?
    a) Phrenic nerves and common cardinal veins
    b) Developing heart and lungs
    c) Pericardial cavity and diaphragm
    d) Diaphragm and mediastinum

101. The musculature of the diaphragm originates from myoblasts in which somites?
    a) Cervical and thoraco-abdominal somites
    b) Thoracic and lumbar somites
    c) Sacral and coccygeal somites
    d) Only thoraco-abdominal somites

102. Where do myoblasts from the caudal cervical somites migrate during diaphragm development?
    a) Into the pericardial cavity
    b) Into the septum transversum
    c) Into the thoracic cavity
    d) Into the developing abdominal muscles

103. Which spinal nerves innervate the musculature of the central region of the diaphragm?
    a) Ventral branches of thoracic spinal nerves
    b) Ventral branches of lumbar spinal nerves
    c) Ventral branches of caudal cervical nerves
    d) Dorsal branches of cervical nerves

104. The central region of the diaphragm is innervated by which nerve?
    a) Sciatic nerve b) Phrenic nerve
    c) Vagus nerve d) Pectoral nerve

105. Which part of the diaphragm is innervated by ventral branches of thoracic and lumbar spinal nerves?
    a) The central region
    b) The muscular rim of the diaphragm
    c) The aortic hiatus
    d) The pericardial cavity

106. What structure passes through the aortic hiatus of the diaphragm?
    a) Aorta, azygos vein, and thoracic duct b) Oesophagus and vagus nerves
    c) Caudal vena cava d) Phrenic nerves

107. The oesophageal hiatus allows passage of which structures?
   a) Aorta and azygos vein
   b) Oesophagus and vagus nerves
   c) Caudal vena cava
   d) Thoracic duct and phrenic nerves

108. Which structure passes through the caval foramen of the diaphragm?
   a) Oesophagus b) Aorta
   c) Caudal vena cava d) Thoracic duct

109. The phrenic nerves are formed by ventral branches of which spinal nerves?
   a) Thoracic and lumbar nerves b) Cervical and thoracic nerves
   c) Caudal cervical nerves d) Sacral and coccygeal nerves

110. What is the primary function of the diaphragm's muscular rim?
   a) To assist in the expansion of the lungs
   b) To separate the thoracic and abdominal cavities
   c) To support the pericardium
   d) To provide a structure for the pleural cavities

111. Congenital diaphragmatic herniation occurs due to:
   a) Overdevelopment of the pleuro-peritoneal folds
   b) Failure of the embryonic diaphragm components to unite and form a complete partition
   c) Excessive growth of the mesoesophagus
   d) Abnormal growth of the peritoneum

112. What condition results when abdominal viscera pass through a persistent opening between the abdominal and thoracic cavities?
   a) Diaphragmatic atrophy
   b) Congenital diaphragmatic herniation
   c) Abdominal perforation
   d) Thoracic enlargement

113. Which type of congenital diaphragmatic herniation is the most common in humans?
   a) Peritoneal-pericardial herniation b) Pleuro-peritoneal herniation
   c) Abdominal hernia d) Cardiac herniation

114. Pleuro-peritoneal herniation occurs due to:
   a) Failure of the septum transversum to develop
   b) Incomplete fusion of the pleuro-peritoneal folds
   c) Overdevelopment of the pericardial cavity
   d) Abnormal lateral body folding

115. In pleuro-peritoneal herniation, the defect usually occurs on which side of the body?
   a) Right side b) Left side
   c) Both sides equally d) Center of the body

116. What is the most common abdominal viscera involved in pleuro-peritoneal herniation in humans?

a) Liver and intestines
b) Stomach and intestines
c) Liver and stomach
d) Heart and lungs

117. Peritoneal-pericardial herniation is more common in which species?

a) Humans and primates
b) Dogs and cats
c) Horses and cows
d) Birds and reptiles

118. What causes peritoneal-pericardial herniation?

a) Failure of the mesoesophagus to develop
b) Defect in the development of the septum transversum
c) Excessive fusion of the peritoneum
d) Incomplete formation of the pleuro-peritoneal folds

119. Which abdominal viscera are commonly involved in peritoneal-pericardial herniation in domestic animals?

a) Liver and intestines
b) Pyloric region of the stomach and intestines
c) Kidneys and spleen
d) Pancreas and lungs

120. Which factor contributes to the development of peritoneal-pericardial herniation?

a) Incomplete fusion of the thoracic wall during lateral body folding
b) Overdevelopment of the pleuro-peritoneal folds
c) Excessive closure of the pleuro-peritoneal canals
d) Failure of the stomach to rotate properly

121. The lateral folding of the body wall results in the formation of which structures?

a) Left and right intra-embryonic coeloms
b) Peritoneum and mesenteries
c) Ventral and dorsal body walls
d) Pleural and pericardial cavities

122. The gut is initially suspended by folds of which type of mesoderm?

a) Somatic mesoderm
b) Extra-embryonic mesoderm
c) Splanchnic mesoderm
d) Ectoderm

123. What is the mesothelium lining the abdominal cavity referred to as?

a) Endoderm
b) Peritoneum
c) Pleura
d) Pericardium

124. Early in its development, the gut is attached to the body wall by:

a) A single layer of mesoderm
b) Dorsal and ventral mesenteries
c) Only dorsal mesenteries
d) Only ventral mesenteries

125. The atrophy of the ventral mesentery allows the gut to:
   a) Increase in length and undergo partial rotation
   b) Become retro-peritoneal
   c) Connect to the thoracic cavity
   d) Form the left and right vaginal processes
126. What does the atrophy of the ventral mesentery result in?
   a) Coalescence of the left and right coelomic cavities
   b) Formation of the diaphragm
   c) Fusion of the stomach and intestines
   d) Formation of the pleuro-pericardial folds
127. Which of the following statements is correct regarding the peritoneal cavity?
   a) It contains a large amount of fluid for organ movement
   b) It is a large cavity where all abdominal organs are located
   c) It normally contains only a thin film of peritoneal fluid of mesothelial origin
   d) It is only present in humans
128. The term 'omentum' refers to:
   a) A ligament that attaches the liver to the diaphragm
   b) A fold of peritoneum that attaches an organ to the stomach
   c) A structure that connects the stomach to the intestines
   d) A layer of mesoderm surrounding the abdominal cavity
129. The dorsal and ventral folds of peritoneum that suspend and anchor the stomach are called:
   a) Dorsal and ventral mesogastrium
   b) Greater and lesser omentum
   c) Peritoneal ligaments
   d) Mesenteries
130. During rotation of the stomach to the left, the dorsal mesogastrium:
   a) Becomes the falciform ligament
   b) Elongates and is drawn to the left, forming the omental bursa
   c) Forms the lesser omentum
   d) Does not change in position
131. The greater omentum consists of:
   a) A single fold of peritoneum
   b) Two leaves: superficial and deep folds of peritoneum
   c) A fold of peritoneum attaching the liver to the diaphragm
   d) A pouch that encloses the spleen
132. The spleen develops from mesodermal aggregations within which part of the greater omentum?
   a) Deep leaf
   b) Superficial leaf
   c) Falciform ligament
   d) Lesser omentum

133. The dorsal bud of the pancreas extends into which part of the greater omentum?
   a) Superficial fold b) Deep fold
   c) mental bursa d) Lesser omentum
134. The lesser omentum forms from the modification of the ventral mesogastrium due to the developing:
   a) Spleen b) Pancreas
   c) Liver d) Kidney
135. The coelom, located outside the embryonic disc is referred to as
   a) Extra embryonic coelom or exocoelom b) Intra embryonic coelom
   c) Chrion d) Amnion
136. _______________ gives rise to the visceral portions of the peritoneum and pleura)
   a) Somatic mesoderm b) Visceral mesoderm
   c) Trophoectoderm d) Rauber's layer
137. The intra embryonic mesoderm is established in
   a) A posterior to anterior direction b) An anterior to posterior direction
   c) A medial to lateral direction d) A lateral to medial direction
138. _______________is continuous with the extra-embryonic mesoderm.
   a) Paraxial mesoderm b) Intermediate mesoderm
   c) Lateral mesoderm d) All of the above

Answer Key

1	b	2	a	3	c	4	a	5	a	6	d	7	a
8	b	9	a	10	d	11	a	12	a	13	b	14	c
15	a	16	b	17	a	18	c	19	d	20	b	21	c
22	c	23	c	24	c	25	b	26	b	27	b	28	d
29	a	30	b	31	d	32	d	33	d	34	d	35	b
36	b	37	c	38	b	39	c	40	b	41	b	42	c
43	c	44	c	45	c	46	a	47	b	48	c	49	c
50	c	51	b	52	d	53	d	54	d	55	b	56	c
57	c	58	c	59	b	60	b	61	c	62	c	63	c
64	a	65	b	66	c	67	c	68	b	69	c	70	a
71	b	72	b	73	c	74	c	75	c	76	b	77	b
78	b	79	b	80	c	81	a	82	a	83	b	84	a
85	b	86	b	87	b	88	a	89	c	90	b	91	d
92	b	93	c	94	a	95	a	96	d	97	b	98	c
99	b	100	a	101	a	102	b	103	c	104	b	105	b
106	a	107	b	108	c	109	c	110	b	111	b	112	b
113	b	114	b	115	b	116	b	117	b	118	b	119	b
120	a	121	a	122	c	123	b	124	b	125	a	126	a
127	c	128	b	129	a	130	b	131	b	132	b	133	a
134	c	135	a	136	b	137	a	138	c				

12

Development of Fetal Membranes

Dayanidhi Jena[1], Priyanka Narwade[2], Vinod Kumar[1] and Tanmoy Rana[3]

[1]*Teaching Veterinary Clinical Complex, Faculty of Veterinary & Animal Sciences, Institute of Agricultural Sciences, Banaras Hindu University, Banaras, Uttar Pradesh*

[2]*Department of Veterinary Gynaecology & Obstetrics, Faculty of Veterinary & Animal Sciences, Institute of Agricultural Sciences, Banaras Hindu University, Banaras, Uttar Pradesh*

[3]*Department of Veterinary Clinical Complex, West Bengal University of Aniaml & Fishery Sciences, Kolkata, West Bengal*

Introduction

The mammalian embryos are subdivided into two groups namely domestic animals where extraembryonic membranes form by folding process, and primates where blastocyst implants very soon after it enters the uterus and extra embryonic membranes forms after implantations. The major function of fetal membranes is to provide nutrients to developing fetus, protection, synthesis of enzymes and hormones and caring of fetal waste products. It is consisted of yolk sac, amnion, allantoic and trophoblast or chorion. The trophoblast is the single most important tissue of fetal membranes which has potential role in absorbing, transmitting and handling nutritive and waste products.

Yolk sac

It is a primitive structure. Develops early in the embryonic period from the entoderm which disappears after short period of time in ruminants. The uterine milk, secreted by the endometrial glands, is absorbed by the blastocyst along with yolk sac to provide nutrition to early embryo. Before forming other embryonic membranes yolk sac performs limited functions whose role is limited during mid and late gestation.

Amnion

It is an ectodermic vesicle that arises from an out folding of the chorion which is a double walled sac that completely surrounds the fetus except at the umbilical ring. The inner layer of this double-walled sac is the "true amnion" and the outer layer is the "false amnion" amnion chorion. Like yolk sac, the amnion chorion also lasts for shorter period.The amniotic fluid is clear, colorless and mucous in nature.

Source of amniotic fluid: In early to mid-gestation, it is probably from the amniotic epithelium and from fetal urine as the fluid is quite watery. As gestation advances, the allantoic fluid increase in volume while the amniotic fluid volume remains fairly static but becomes viscid and glairy because the bladder sphincter prevents further release of urine in to the amniotic cavity. The probable source of mucous amniotic fluid is then the secretions of the nasopharynx and saliva of the fetus.

The amniotic fluid serves multiple functions as it is bactericidal and prevents adhesions to embryonic skin and the amniotic membrane. In addition to that. it also helps in the initial steps of implantation when the expanding chorionic sac is brought in to close apposition with the endometrium. Furthermore, it provides a watery medium in which the embryo can develop free from distortions that would arise from being pressed against rigid surrounding structures.

Amount of amniotic fluid towards the end of gestation

Species	*Amount (ml)*
Cow	2000-8000
Mare	3000-7000
Goat	400-1200
Ewe	350-750
Sow	40-200
Dogs and cats	8-30

Allantoic

It arises during the second or third week of gestation in bovine fetuses as an out pocketing of the hind gut and consists of endoderm covered by vascular layer of splanchnopleuric mesoderm.

As the Allantois grows and enlarges, it extends between the true and false amnion. The outer layer of the Allantoic fuses with the trophoblast, false amnion, or serosa to form the chorioallantois. The allantois fluid is clear, watery, amber coloured and contains albumen, fructose and urea.

Source of allantoic fluid: Allantoic cavity stores the waste products of the fetal kidneys, which pass to it from the bladder through the umbilical cord by means of the urachus.

Amount of allantoic fluid towards the end of gestation.

Species	*Amount (ml)*
Cow	4000-15,000
Mare	8000-18000
Sheep, Goat	500-1500
Sow	100-200
Dog	10-50
Cat	3-15

Multiple Choice Questions

1. Which of the following structure is derived from Trophoblastic cells?

   a) Amnion b) Chorion

   c) Yolk sac d) Allontoic

2. In which of the following species, Blastocyst is filamentous?
   a) Ewe, Sow, Cow
   b) Mare, Doe, Ewe
   c) Buffalo, Doe, Ewe
   d) Sow, Mare, Ewe
3. Blastocyst is spherical in which of the following species?
   a) Cow
   b) Mare
   c) Buffalo
   d) Sow
4. Yolk sac develops from _______________?
   a) Endoderm
   b) Primitive endoderm
   c) Mare
   d) Ewe
5. In which of the following species, amniotic proliferation is observed?
   a) Mare
   b) Ewe
   c) Cow
   d) Both a and b
6. __________________ prevents adhesion of embryonic skin to uterine tissue.
   a) Amnion
   b) Allontois
   c) Chorion
   d) Chorio-allontois
7. What are the characteristics features of allantoic fluid?
   a) Clear, Watery, Amber
   b) Transperant, Mucoid, Thick
   c) Opaque, Clear, Amber
   d) Mucoid, Clear, Amber
8. What are the characteristics of amniotic fluid?
   a) Mucoid, Thick, Brown
   b) Clear, Colourless , Mucoid
   c) Mucoid, Clear, Amber
   d) Clear, Watery, Amber
9. Which of the following fetal membrane develops after 13-15 weeks of conception in cow ?
   a) Yolk sac
   b) Allantois
   c) Chorion
   d) Amnion
10. The fluid filled sac that collect major amount of liquid waste from the embryo______.
    a) Allantois
    b) Amnion
    c) Chorioallantois
    d) chorion
11. The .... membrane is the fetal contribution to the placenta and it provides the surface for attachment to the endometrium.
    a) Chorion
    b) Amnion
    c) Allantois
    d) Alanto-chorion
12. A small, irregular shaped, white, elevated epithelial thickening observed on amniotic sac is termed as _______________.
    a) Hippomenes
    b) Amniotic plaque
    c) Amniotic sand
    d) Both b and c
13. Allantoic fluid contains amorphous, semisolid amber coloured, soft, pliable, rubber like, irregular shaped masses known as __________________.
    a) Hippomanes
    b) Amniotic plaque
    c) Amniotic sand
    d) Both b and c

14. Allantoic calculi are also referred as __________________.
    a) Amniotic plaque b) Amniotic sand
    c) Hippomanes d) None of the above
15. Hippomanes observed generally in which species?
    a) Cow, Ewe b) Doe
    c) Sow d) All of the above
16. Amount of amniotic fluid present towards the end of gestation in cattle is ________.
    a) 2000-8000 ml b) 3000- 7000 ml
    c) 500-1000 ml d) 400-1200 ml
17. In cattle, excessive accumulation of foetal fluids can occasionally occur in either the amniotic or allantoic sacs. This condition is referred to as ______________.
    a) Hydrops of the fetal sacs b) Fetal Ascites
    c) Anasarca d) Oedema
18. Calculi are found in the allantoic fluid in a number of species. In the mare, these calculi, which occur as small brown masses up to 4 cm in diameter, are referred to as___________.
    a) Hippomanes b) Chorionic Calculi
    c) Amniotic Calculi d) Yolk Sac Calculi
19. The term ____ is used to describe the embryo or fetus and associated fluid-filled membranes
    a) Conceptus b) Foetus
    c) Embryonated mass d) Blastula
20. The separation of somatopleure into an inner _______which surrounds the embryo, and an outer ___________ layer.
    a) Amnion chorion. b) Chorion amnion
    c) Allantois amnion d) Allantois chorion
21. In domestic animals, which fetal membrane develops as a diverticulum of the hindgut?
    a) Allantois b) Amnion
    c) Chorion d) Yolk sac
22. Which of the following fetal membrane vascularizes the chorion?
    a) Allantois b) Amnion
    c) Yolk sac d) Vitelline duct
23. Which layer of the fetal membrane serves as a reservoir for metabolic waste products?
    a) Allantois b) Amnion
    c) Yolk sac d) Vitelline duct
24. In viviparous animals, which of the following structure forms as a result of apposition of the fetal membranes to uterine tissue?
    a) Placenta b) Chorioamniotic raphé
    c) Umblicus d) Allantoic sac

25. The extra-embryonic or fetal membranes of domestic mammals, consisting of yolk sac, amnion, chorion and allantois, develop in a manner similar to those of______.
    a) Birds. b) Reptile
    c) Amphibian d) Avian

26. In …., fetal membranes are involved in hormone production and formation of the placenta)
    a) Mammals b) Reptile
    c) Amphibian d) Avian

27. Structures or tissues which develop from the zygote and are of functional importance only in embryonic life which do not form part of the embryo itself are called as______________.
    a) Extra-embryonic or foetal membranes.
    b) Amniotic fold
    c) Chorioallantoic fold
    d) Embryonic disc

28. The ______________is composed of extra-embryonic splanchnopleure and is connected to the embryonic midgut via the vitelline duct.
    a) Allantois b) Amnion
    c) Chorion d) Yolk sac

29. What is the primary function of amniotic fluid in bovine fetuses?
    a) Nutrient transport b) Shock absorption
    c) Hormone production d) Waste removal

30. Which structure produces amniotic fluid in bovines?
    a) Allantois b) Amnion
    c) Chorion d) Yolk sac

31. What is the main component of amniotic fluid?
    a) Protein b) Lipid
    c) Water d) Carbohydrates

32. What is the primary purpose of the allantoic fluid?
    a) Protection of the fetus b) Storage of waste products
    c) Nutritional support d) Facilitating lung development

33. During which stage of gestation does amniotic fluid volume peak in bovines?
    a) Early gestation b) Mid gestation
    c) Late gestation d) At parturition

34. What fetal membrane forms the interface with maternal tissues?
    a) Amnion b) Allantois
    c) Chorion d) Yolk sac

35. Which fetal membrane is responsible for gas exchange in bovines?
    a) Amnion b) Chorion
    c) Allantois d) Yolk sac

36. How does the composition of allantoic fluid differ from amniotic fluid?
    a) Higher protein content
    b) Higher electrolyte concentration
    c) Lower water content
    d) More nutrients
37. What is the primary source of fetal urine in bovines?
    a) Amniotic fluid
    b) Allantoic fluid
    c) Fetal kidneys
    d) Maternal blood
38. What role does the chorion play in fetal development?
    a) Provides nutrients
    b) Forms the placenta
    c) Produces hormones
    d) Stores waste
39. At what stage of gestation does the chorion become fully vascularized?
    a) First trimester
    b) Mid gestation
    c) Late gestation
    d) Just before parturition
40. What happens to amniotic fluid volume as the pregnancy progresses?
    a) Decreases steadily
    b) Increases steadily
    c) Remains constant
    d) Fluctuates randomly
41. Which fetal membrane helps to anchor the placenta to the uterus?
    a) Amnion
    b) Allantois
    c) Chorion
    d) Yolk sac
42. What is a common cause of excessive amniotic fluid (hydramnios) in bovines?
    a) Maternal dehydration
    b) Fetal anomalies
    c) Inadequate nutrition
    d) Normal variation
43. Which hormone is primarily produced by the placenta in bovines?
    a) Progesterone
    b) Estrogen
    c) Relaxin
    d) Human chorionic gonadotropin
44. What is the significance of the umbilical cord in fetal development?
    a) Provides protection
    b) Facilitates nutrient and waste exchange
    c) Maintains fluid balance
    d) Produces hormones
45. How does fetal movement affect amniotic fluid levels?
    a) Increases fluid volume
    b) Decreases fluid volume
    c) Has no effect
    d) Alters fluid composition
46. which of the following conditions may arise from a ruptured amniotic sac?
    a) Infection
    b) Hydramnios
    c) Premature labor
    d) Both a and c
47. During what time of the gestation, the allantois forms?
    a) Second to third week
    b) Fourth to fifth week
    c) Sixth to seventh week
    d) After tenth week

48. Which fetal membrane is primarily involved in protecting the fetus from mechanical injury?
    a) Amnion b) Allantois
    c) Chorion d) Yolk sac
49. what are the functions of the fetal membrane?
    a) Transferring of nutrients from dam to fetus.
    b) Gaseous exchange
    c) Fetal waste management.
    d) All of the above.
50. The allantois is formed completely at around what stage of gestation?
    a) 10-15 days. b) 25 to 30 days.
    c) 60 to 90 days. d) 120 days to 150 days
51. What are the function of trophoblast layer of fetal membrane?
    a) Absorbing of nutrient. b) Transmitting the waste product.
    c) Erosive action on endometrium. d) All of these.
52. The waste products from fetal kidney are stored mainly in_______.
    a) Amniotic cavity. b) Allantoic Cavity.
    c) Foetal intestine. d) None of above.
53. Calcium precipitation in allantochorion starts at what stage of gestation?
    a) 30-50 days b) 60-90 days
    c) 120-150 days d) None of the above
54. In which of the following species hippomanes are not found?
    a) Dog b) Cow
    c) Ewe d) Sow
55. Amnion formation occur at which days of gestational life of ewe and cow?
    a) 1-2 b) 7-10
    c) 13-16 d) 20-25
56. Mottling or white streaking is observed in which fetal membrane?
    a) Chorion b) Allantois
    c) Amnion d) None of the above.
57. Necrotic tips of chorioallantois is found in which of the following species?
    a) Cow b) Sheep
    c) Sow d) All of the above
58. Amniotic plaques are most noticeable during which stage of gestation?
    a) During 1-3 month b) Between 3 to 5 months
    c) Between 3-7 months d) Throughout the gestation
59. Amount of amniotic fluid present at the end of gestation of cow and mare respectively
    a) 2000-8000 and 3000-7000 b) 1000-5000 and 2000- 3000
    c) 3000-4000 and 4000-5000 d) 2000-8000 and 8000-10000.

60. Cervical star present over the internal os of the Cervix in which of the following species?
   a) Mare b) Bitch
   c) Cow d) Sow

61. Allantoic fluid and amniotic fluid are also called ________ and ________ respectively.
   a) 1st water bag and 2nd water bag b) 2nd water bag and 1st water bag
   c) 3rd water bag and 1 St water bag. d) 2nd water bag and 3rd water bag

62. The allantois is attached to various points of amnion in which of the following species?
   a) Cow b) Ewe
   c) Sow d) All of the above

63. The Chorion and amnion are derived from which of the following structure?
   a) Somatopleure b) Splanchanopleure
   c) Both d) None of the above

64. Allantois and yolk sac are derived from which structure?
   a) Splanchanopleure b) Somatopleure
   c) Both d) None of the above

65. In which of the following species fetus floats freely in allantoic cavity?
   a) Dog b) Cat
   c) Horse d) All of the above

66. Which of following fetal membrane act as embryonic urinary bladder?
   a) Allantois b) Amnion
   c) Chorion d) Yolk sac

67. in mare and sow which type of placentation is observed?
   a) Diffuse b) Cotyledonary
   c) Multiplex d) Zonary

68. Zonary type of placentation is observed in which of the following animal?
   a) Dog b) Mare
   c) Cow d) Ewe

69. Areolae in placenta are more abundant in which of the following specie?
   a) Mare b) Cow
   c) Sow d) Bitch

70. Cotyledonary placenta is found in which of the following animals?
   a) Ruminants b) Equine
   c) Canine and feline d) Rodents

71. Multiplex type of placentation is also known as ____________.
   a) Diffuse b) Cotyledonary
   c) Discoidal d) Zonary

72. In some disease conditions, primitive placental structures develop between allantois-chorion and endometrium which is known as ________________.

a) Adventitious placenta or accessory placentomes
b) Diffuse placenta
c) Zonary placenta
d) Discoidal discs

73. The structure arising from fusion of maternal caruncle and fetal cotyledon are termed as____.

a) Uterine sand b) Amniotic sand
c) Hippomanes d) Placentomes

74. Zonary placenta is found in which of the following animals?

a) Ruminants b) Equine
c) Canine and feline d) Rodents

75. Discoidal type placenta is found in which of the following animals?

a) Ruminants b) Equine
c) Canine and feline d) Primates and rodents

76. Placental hematomas or extravasations are brown in colour in which species?

a) Ruminants b) Equine
c) Feline d) Canine

77. Placental hematomas or extravasations are green in colour in which species?

a) Ruminants b) Equine
c) Feline d) Canine

78. Syndesmochorial type placentation is found in which of the following species?

a) Ruminants b) Equine
c) Feline d) Canine

79. In syndesmochorial type placentation, which layer is absent?

a) Endothelium b) Connective tissues
c) Trophoblast d) Maternal epithelium

80. In canine and felines which of the following placentation is observed?

a) Epitheliochorial b) Endotheiliochorial
c) Hemochorial d) Syndesmochorial

81. Hemochorial placentation is found in ____________.

a) Ruminants b) Equine
c) Feline d) Human and rodents

82. All maternal tissues are absent in which type of placentation?

a) Epitheliochorial b) Endotheiliochorial
c) Hemochorial d) Syndesmochorial

83. The deciduate or conjoined type of placentation is found in which of the following animal?

a) Rodent b) Human

c) Canine d) All of the above

84. The indeciduate or apposed type placentation is observed in which animals?

a) Ruminants b) Swine

c) Horses d) All of the above

85. The endothelium lies in a "lake or pool of maternal blood" in which type of placentation?

a) Epitheliochorial b) Endotheiliochorial

c) Hemochorial d) Syndesmochorial

Answer Key

1	b	2	a	3	b	4	b	5	d	6	a	7	a
8	b	9	d	10	a	11	d	12	d	13	a	14	c
15	d	16	a	17	a	18	a	19	a	20	a	21	a
22	a	23	a	24	a	25	a	26	a	27	a	28	d
29	b	30	b	31	c	32	b	33	c	34	c	35	b
36	b	37	c	38	b	39	c	40	b	41	c	42	b
43	a	44	b	45	c	46	d	47	a	48	a	49	d
50	b	51	d	52	b	53	b	54	a	55	c	56	b
57	a	58	c	59	a	60	a	61	a	62	d	63	a
64	a	65	d	66	a	67	a	68	a	69	c	70	a
71	b	72	a	73	d	74	c	75	d	76	c	77	d
78	a	79	d	80	b	81	d	82	c	83	d	84	d
85	c												

13

Implantation and Placentation and Foetal Circulation

Dangeti V.V.N. Durga Prasad[1], M.P.S Tomar[2], Avinash Palli[3] and K. Archana[2]

[1]*Section of Veterinary Anatomy, ICAR-IVRI, Izatnagar, Bareilly-243122, Uttar Pradesh*
[2]*NTR Veterinary Sciences College, Gannavaram, S.V.V.U., Andhra Pradesh*
[3]*School of Veterinary and Animal Science, CUTM, Paralakhemundi, Odisha*

Introduction

Reproduction involves the intricate interplay of physiological processes to ensure the successful growth and development of the embryo and fetus. Three key processes—implantation, placentation, and the establishment of fetal circulation—are fundamental to a viable pregnancy. These stages ensure the fetus receives adequate nutrients, oxygen, and support for development. Below is a detailed elaboration of each process.

1. Implantation

Implantation is the process by which the blastocyst (a hollow structure formed in the early development of mammals) embeds itself into the uterine wall. It is the first critical step in establishing a pregnancy.

Phases of Implantation

1. Apposition: The blastocyst loosely attaches to the endometrium (the inner lining of the uterus).
2. Adhesion: The trophoblast cells (outer layer of the blastocyst) firmly attach to the uterine lining.
3. Invasion: The trophoblast differentiates into two layers:

Cytotrophoblast: The inner cellular layer that serves as the proliferative zone.

Syncytiotrophoblast: The outer multinucleated layer that invades the endometrium, facilitating deeper embedding.

Significance

Implantation typically occurs 6–10 days after fertilization.

It ensures the establishment of an early connection between the embryo and maternal blood supply.

Successful implantation depends on hormonal regulation, especially the roles of estrogen and progesterone, which prepare the endometrium to be receptive.

2. Placentation

Placentation refers to the formation and maturation of the placenta, the critical organ that serves as the interface between the mother and fetus.

Structure of the Placenta:

1. Maternal Component: The decidua basalis forms the maternal contribution to the placenta)
2. Fetal Component: The chorionic villi, derived from the trophoblast, develop into intricate structures that interact with maternal blood)

Functions of the Placenta

Nutrient Exchange: The placenta transports glucose, amino acids, and fatty acids to the fetus.

Gas Exchange: It facilitates oxygen uptake and carbon dioxide removal between maternal and fetal blood)

Waste Elimination: Fetal metabolic waste products like urea and creatinine are transferred to maternal blood for excretion.

Endocrine Role: Produces essential hormones, such as:

hCG (human chorionic gonadotropin): Supports the corpus luteum.

Progesterone: Maintains uterine quiescence.

Estrogen: Stimulates uterine and fetal growth.

Immunological Barrier: Protects the fetus from maternal immune attack while allowing limited antibody transfer for passive immunity.

Timeline:

By the end of the first trimester, the placenta is fully developed and functional, continuing to grow throughout pregnancy.

3. Fetal Circulation

Fetal circulation is a specialized system that supports life in utero by connecting the fetus to the placenta via the umbilical cord)It enables the fetus to obtain oxygen and nutrients and to dispose of waste products, bypassing the non-functional fetal lungs and liver.

Key Features of Fetal Circulation

1. Umbilical Cord: Contains:Two umbilical arteries: Carry deoxygenated blood and waste from the fetus to the placenta)One umbilical vein: Carries oxygenated blood and nutrients from the placenta to the fetus.
2. Specialized Pathways:Ductus Venosus: Shunts oxygenated blood from the umbilical vein to the inferior vena cava, bypassing the liver.

Foramen Ovale: An opening between the right and left atria, allowing oxygen-rich blood to bypass the lungs and flow directly to the systemic circulation.

Ductus Arteriosus: Connects the pulmonary artery to the descending aorta, diverting blood from the pulmonary circuit.

Postnatal Adaptation

At birth, the transition from fetal to newborn circulation occurs rapidly as the baby takes its first breath. This leads to:

Closure of the foramen ovale.

Functional closure of the ductus arteriosus and ductus venosus.

The establishment of independent pulmonary and systemic circulation.

Significance

These adaptations ensure optimal oxygen delivery during fetal life while preparing the newborn for survival in an external environment.

Implantation, placentation, and fetal circulation are interdependent processes essential for the sustenance of fetal life. Implantation anchors the embryo to the uterus, while placentation establishes a vital support system to nurture the fetus. Simultaneously, fetal circulation ensures efficient nutrient and gas transport through a specialized vascular system. These stages exemplify the delicate coordination required for the development of new life. Understanding these processes provides critical insights into normal and pathological pregnancy.

Multiple Choice Questions

1. What is the primary site for embryo implantation in humans?
   a) Ovary b) Fallopian tube
   c) Uterine lining d) Cervix
2. What hormone is primarily responsible for preparing the uterine lining for implantation?
   a) Estrogen b) Progesterone
   c) Testosterone d) Insulin
3. How long after fertilization does the embryo typically reach the uterus?
   a) 3 days b) 5 days
   c) 7 days d) 14 days
4. What is the name of the process where the embryo embeds itself into the uterine lining?
   a) Fertilization b) Implantation
   c) Ovulation d) Gastrulation
5. Which part of the embryo makes direct contact with the uterine lining during implantation?
   a) Blastocyst b) Morula
   c) Zygote d) Oocyte
6. Which structure helps the embryo adhere to the uterine wall?
   a) Placenta b) Chorion
   c) Trophoblast d) Amnion

7. What is the name of the stage of the embryo that is typically implanted into the uterine lining?
   a) Morula b) Blastocyst
   c) Zygote d) Gastrula
8. When does the implantation process typically begin?
   a) During ovulation b) Immediately after fertilization
   c) 6-7 days after fertilization d) 14 days after fertilization
9. What does the trophoblast eventually develop into?
   a) Placenta b) Amnion
   c) Umbilical cord d) Yolk sac
10. What is the role of the endometrium in embryo implantation?
   a) Providing nutrients b) Protecting the embryo
   c) Allowing the embryo to attach d) Producing hormones
11. Which phase of the menstrual cycle is most receptive to implantation?
   a) Follicular phase b) Ovulatory phase
   c) Luteal phase d) Menstrual phase
12. What is the name of the fluid-filled cavity in the blastocyst that eventually forms the amniotic sac?
   a) Blastocoel b) Amniotic cavity
   c) Chorionic cavity d) Yolk sac
13. What cells are responsible for forming the placenta?
   a) Epiblast cells b) Hypoblast cells
   c) Trophoblast cells d) Mesoderm cells
14. Which hormone is produced by the embryo to signal pregnancy to the mother?
   a) Human chorionic gonadotropin (hCG) b) Luteinizing hormone (LH)
   c) Follicle-stimulating hormone (FSH) d) Estrogen
15. What is the function of the syncytiotrophoblast?
   a) Producing hormones b) Facilitating embryo attachment
   c) Invading the uterine lining d) Forming the amniotic sac
16. What occurs during the process of decidualization?
   a) The embryo detaches from the uterus
   b) The endometrial lining transforms to support the embryo
   c) The trophoblast forms the placenta
   d) The embryo reaches the blastocyst stage
17. Which structure provides nutrients to the developing embryo before the placenta forms?
   a) Yolk sac b) Amniotic sac
   c) Umbilical cord d) Chorion

18. What is the typical duration of the implantation window?
    a) 1-2 days
    b) 3-4 days
    c) 5-7 days
    d) 10-14 days
19. What role does the chorion play in early pregnancy?
    a) It forms the amniotic sac
    b) It produces the hCG hormone
    c) It forms the primary umbilical blood vessels
    d) It helps in the formation of the embryo's skeleton
20. When does the embryo start producing its own hCG?
    a) Immediately after fertilization
    b) After implantation
    c) At the end of the first trimester
    d) Just before birth
21. How does the maternal immune system respond to the presence of the embryo?
    a) By rejecting the embryo
    b) By becoming more active
    c) By tolerating the embryo
    d) By forming a barrier around the embryo
22. What is the name of the condition where the embryo implants outside the uterine cavity?
    a) Ectopic pregnancy
    b) Miscarriage
    c) Molar pregnancy
    d) Placental abruption
23. Which part of the blastocyst will eventually become the embryo proper?
    a) Trophoblast
    b) Inner cell mass
    c) Blastocoel
    d) Cytotrophoblast
24. What triggers the transition from the luteal phase to early pregnancy?
    a) Increased progesterone levels
    b) Decreased estrogen levels
    c) Presence of hCG in the bloodstream
    d) Ovulation
25. What type of tissue does the decidua refer to?
    a) The outer layer of the embryo
    b) The uterine lining during pregnancy
    c) The placenta
    d) The amniotic membrane
26. Which process involves the breakdown of the maternal blood vessels for embryo nourishment?
    a) Decidualization
    b) Trophoblastic invasion
    c) Placental separation
    d) Amniotic fluid formation
27. What is the primary function of the amniotic fluid?
    a) Providing nutrients
    b) Protecting the embryo from physical trauma

c) Transporting waste
d) Stimulating uterine contractions

28. When does the formation of the placenta typically begin?
a) During fertilization
b) Immediately after implantation
c) At the end of the first trimester
d) During the second trimester

29. Which structure becomes part of the umbilical cord?
a) Amniotic sac
b) Yolk sac
c) Allantois
d) Chorionic villi

30. What is the role of the cytotrophoblast in implantation?
a) To invade the uterine lining
b) To form the outer layer of the placenta
c) To provide nutrients to the embryo
d) To produce hormones

31. How does the embryo prevent the maternal immune system from rejecting it?
a) By secreting immunosuppressive factors
b) By hiding from the immune system
c) By promoting inflammation
d) By increasing hCG levels

32. What is the role of the trophoblast in the formation of the placenta?
a) It forms the embryo's organs
b) It develops into the placenta and supports the embryo
c) It creates the amniotic fluid
d) It forms the umbilical cord

33. Which of the following best describes the implantation site in the endometrium?
a) Fundus
b) Corpus
c) Cervix
d) Uterine lining

34. What is the significance of the hCG hormone in early pregnancy tests?
a) It indicates ovulation
b) It confirms successful embryo implantation
c) It measures progesterone levels
d) It tracks fetal development

35. How does the embryo's blastocyst stage impact its implantation process?
a) It helps the embryo move through the fallopian tube
b) It facilitates the embryo's attachment to the uterine lining
c) It starts the development of the umbilical cord
d) It prevents early miscarriage

36. What happens if implantation does not occur successfully?
a) The embryo continues to develop normally
b) The embryo is expelled from the uterus

c) The embryo undergoes ectopic development

d) The pregnancy continues with no issues

37. Which cells in the blastocyst will form the embryo and its supporting structures?

a) Inner cell mass b) Trophoblast cells

c) Cytotrophoblast cells d) Epiblast cells

38. What is the primary function of the placenta in mammals?

a) Digestion b) Respiration

c) Nutrient and gas exchange d) Excretion

39. Which structure forms the fetal part of the placenta?

a) Endometrium b) Chorion

c) Myometrium d) Amnion

40. In which species is the placenta described as diffuse?

a) Cattle b) Horses

c) Pigs d) Humans

41. What type of placenta is characterized by a single, central disc of attachment?

a) Diffuse b) Cotyledonary

c) Zonary d) Discoid

42. Which type of placenta is found in humans and rodents?

a) Cotyledonary b) Discoid

c) Zonary d) Diffuse

43. Which fetal membranes contribute to the formation of the placenta?

a) Amnion and allantois b) Chorion and amnion

c) Chorion and allantois d) Yolk sac and chorion

44. What is the name of the placental structure that provides a barrier between maternal and fetal blood?

a) Chorionic villi b) Decidua

c) Amniotic sac d) Umbilical cord

45. Which type of placentation is observed in ruminants like cows and sheep?

a) Discoid b) Cotyledonary

c) Zonary d) Diffuse

46. In which type of placentation does the placenta cover a band around the middle of the fetus?

a) Discoid b) Cotyledonary

c) Zonary d) Diffuse

47. Which type of placenta has multiple localized areas of attachment, each called a cotyledon?

a) Zonary b) Discoid

c) Cotyledonary d) Diffuse

48. The placental barrier in the horse is classified as:
   a) Epitheliochorial b) Endotheliochorial
   c) Syndesmochorial d) Hemochorial
49. In which species is the placenta described as epitheliochorial?
   a) Dogs b) Cattle
   c) Horses d) Humans
50. Which of the following is a key feature of the hemochorial placenta?
   a) Maternal epithelium directly contacts fetal blood
   b) Fetal epithelium directly contacts maternal blood
   c) Maternal and fetal blood remain separate by a thick barrier
   d) There is no direct contact between maternal and fetal blood
51. What structure connects the fetal placenta to the maternal uterus?
   a) Umbilical cord b) Placental disc
   c) Chorionic villi d) Placental artery
52. The placental structure where the maternal and fetal blood vessels are closely opposed is called:
   a) Chorionic villi b) Amniotic sac
   c) Decidua d) Umbilical vein
53. Which type of placenta is classified as having the maternal blood in direct contact with the chorionic epithelium?
   a) Endotheliochorial b) Epitheliochorial
   c) Hemochorial d) Syndesmochorial
54. In which species is the placenta described as syndesmochorial?
   a) Cattle b) Horses
   c) Pigs d) Dogs
55. What is the primary role of the allantois in placentation?
   a) Forming the amniotic cavity b) Supporting nutrient transfer
   c) Collecting metabolic waste d) Developing the chorionic villi
56. Which of the following best describes the cotyledonary placenta?
   a) Single disc-like structure
   b) Multiple cotyledons attached to the caruncles
   c) Band of attachment around the fetus
   d) Whole surface attachment
57. In the diffuse placenta, how is the chorion attached to the endometrium?
   a) Through distinct regions b) Via multiple small areas
   c) Over the entire surface d) Through a central disc
58. The placenta of pigs is typically described as:
   a) Diffuse b) Cotyledonary
   c) Discoid d) Zonary

59. Which placental type involves the chorionic villi being directly bathed by maternal blood?
   a) Epitheliochorial b) Endotheliochorial
   c) Hemochorial d) Syndesmochorial

60. What term describes the maternal tissue that is shed during birth in species with a hemochorial placenta?
   a) Decidua b) Placenta
   c) Amnion d) Chorion

61. Which species has a zonary placenta?
   a) Cattle b) Horses
   c) Dogs d) Pigs

62. Which type of placenta is considered the most invasive and has the least separation between maternal and fetal blood?
   a) Epitheliochorial b) Endotheliochorial
   c) Syndesmochorial d) Hemochorial

63. In which type of placenta does the fetal chorion have direct contact with maternal blood vessels?
   a) Epitheliochorial b) Endotheliochorial
   c) Hemochorial d) Syndesmochorial

64. What is the role of the amniotic fluid?
   a) Nutrient transfer
   b) Protection and cushioning of the fetus
   c) Waste removal
   d) Hormone production

65. The chorion, amnion, allantois, and yolk sac are:
   a) Fetal membranes b) Maternal tissues
   c) Placental hormones d) Amniotic layers

66. The presence of cotyledons is a feature of which placental type?
   a) Discoid b) Zonary
   c) Cotyledonary d) Diffuse

67. Which placental type involves a fusion of the chorionic villi with the endometrial epithelium?
   a) Epitheliochorial b) Endotheliochorial
   c) Syndesmochorial d) Hemochorial

68. In ruminants, the maternal portion of the placenta is known as:
   a) Caruncles b) Cotyledons
   c) Decidua d) Amnion

69. Which structure is responsible for the production of hormones necessary for maintaining pregnancy?
   a) Umbilical cord
   b) Placenta
   c) Amnion
   d) Allantois

70. What is the primary function of the chorionic villi?
   a) Waste removal
   b) Nutrient and gas exchange
   c) Fluid cushioning
   d) Hormone production

71. In the context of placentation, what does 'epitheliochorial' indicate?
   a) Fetal chorionic epithelium is in direct contact with maternal blood
   b) Maternal epithelium is in direct contact with fetal chorionic epithelium
   c) There is a complete separation between maternal and fetal blood
   d) Maternal tissue is fused with fetal tissue

72. What type of placenta involves the maternal uterine epithelium being retained throughout gestation?
   a) Endotheliochorial
   b) Epitheliochorial
   c) Hemochorial
   d) Syndesmochorial

73. The placenta of which animal is classified as discoid?
   a) Sheep
   b) Horse
   c) Human
   d) Dog

74. Which species has a placenta that is primarily diffuse and has a relatively large surface area for maternal-fetal exchange?
   a) Pig
   b) Cow
   c) Cat
   d) Dog

75. What is the primary function of the placenta in fetal circulation?
   a) Oxygenate fetal blood
   b) Filter fetal blood
   c) Produce fetal blood cells
   d) Store fetal blood

76. Which structure allows blood to bypass the fetal liver?
   a) Foramen ovale
   b) Ductus arteriosus
   c) Ductus venosus
   d) Umbilical vein

77. The foramen ovale is located between which two chambers of the heart?
   a) Right atrium and right ventricle
   b) Left atrium and left ventricle
   c) Right atrium and left atrium
   d) Right ventricle and left ventricle

78. Which vessel carries oxygenated blood from the placenta to the fetus?
   a) Umbilical artery
   b) Umbilical vein
   c) Ductus arteriosus
   d) Ductus venosus

79. What happens to the ductus arteriosus after birth?
   a) It becomes the ligamentum arteriosum
   b) It remains open
   c) It becomes the ligamentum venosum
   d) It becomes the umbilical ligament

80. Which structure allows blood to bypass the fetal lungs?
    a) Foramen ovale b) Ductus arteriosus
    c) Ductus venosus d) Umbilical vein
81. The umbilical arteries carry blood from the fetus to the:
    a) Placenta b) Liver
    c) Lungs d) Heart
82. Which of the following is true about fetal hemoglobin?
    a) It has a lower affinity for oxygen than adult hemoglobin
    b) It has a higher affinity for oxygen than adult hemoglobin
    c) It is identical to adult hemoglobin
    d) It is not present in the fetus
83. What is the role of the ductus venosus?
    a) Connects the umbilical vein to the inferior vena cava
    b) Connects the pulmonary artery to the aorta
    c) Connects the right atrium to the left atrium
    d) Connects the umbilical artery to the inferior vena cava
84. Which structure closes shortly after birth to separate the right and left atria?
    a) Foramen ovale b) Ductus arteriosus
    c) Ductus venosus d) Umbilical vein
85. The fetal circulation is designed to:
    a) Maximize oxygen delivery to the lungs
    b) Minimize oxygen delivery to the liver
    c) Maximize oxygen delivery to the brain and heart
    d) Minimize oxygen delivery to the placenta
86. Which vessel carries deoxygenated blood from the fetus to the placenta?
    a) Umbilical artery b) Umbilical vein
    c) Ductus arteriosus d) Ductus venosus
87. What is the primary source of oxygen for the fetus?
    a) Fetal lungs b) Fetal liver
    c) Placenta d) Inferior vena cava
88. Which structure allows blood to flow directly from the right atrium to the left atrium in the fetus?
    a) Foramen ovale b) Ductus arteriosus
    c) Ductus venosus d) Umbilical vein
89. What happens to the foramen ovale after birth?
    a) It becomes the ligamentum arteriosum b) It remains open
    c) It becomes the fossa ovalis d) It becomes the umbilical ligament

90. Which of the following is NOT a feature of fetal circulation?
   a) High pulmonary vascular resistance
   b) Low systemic vascular resistance
   c) Presence of shunts
   d) High oxygen saturation in the umbilical arteries
91. The ductus arteriosus connects which two structures?
   a) Right atrium and left atrium
   b) Pulmonary artery and aorta
   c) Umbilical vein and inferior vena cava
   d) Right ventricle and left ventricle
92. Which structure carries oxygenated blood from the placenta to the fetus?
   a) Umbilical artery b) Umbilical vein
   c) Ductus arteriosus d) Ductus venosus
93. What is the function of the umbilical vein?
   a) Carry deoxygenated blood to the placenta
   b) Carry oxygenated blood to the fetus
   c) Carry deoxygenated blood to the fetus
   d) Carry oxygenated blood to the placenta
94. Which of the following statements about fetal circulation is true?
   a) The fetal lungs are fully functional
   b) The placenta provides oxygen and nutrients to the fetus
   c) The ductus venosus carries blood from the right atrium to the left atrium
   d) The umbilical arteries carry oxygenated blood to the fetus
95. The ductus venosus allows blood to bypass which organ?
   a) Lungs b) Liver
   c) Heart d) Kidneys
96. Which structure closes to form the ligamentum venosum after birth?
   a) Foramen ovale b) Ductus arteriosus
   c) Ductus venosus d) Umbilical vein
97. What is the primary function of the foramen ovale?
   a) Allow blood to bypass the liver
   b) Allow blood to bypass the lungs
   c) Allow blood to bypass the heart
   d) Allow blood to bypass the kidneys
98. Which vessel carries deoxygenated blood from the fetus to the placenta?
   a) Umbilical artery b) Umbilical vein
   c) Ductus arteriosus d) Ductus venosus

99. What happens to the umbilical arteries after birth?
   a) They become the ligamentum arteriosum
   b) They remain open
   c) They become the medial umbilical ligaments
   d) They become the ligamentum venosum

100. Which structure allows blood to bypass the fetal lungs?
   a) Foramen ovale
   b) Ductus arteriosus
   c) Ductus venosus
   d) Umbilical vein

101. The umbilical arteries carry blood from the fetus to the:
   a) Placenta
   b) Liver
   c) Lungs
   d) Heart

102. Which of the following is true about fetal hemoglobin?
   a) It has a lower affinity for oxygen than adult hemoglobin
   b) It has a higher affinity for oxygen than adult hemoglobin
   c) It is identical to adult hemoglobin
   d) It is not present in the fetus

103. What is the role of the ductus venosus?
   a) Connects the umbilical vein to the inferior vena cava
   b) Connects the pulmonary artery to the aorta
   c) Connects the right atrium to the left atrium
   d) Connects the umbilical artery to the inferior vena cava

104. Which structure closes shortly after birth to separate the right and left atria?
   a) Foramen ovale
   b) Ductus arteriosus
   c) Ductus venosus
   d) Umbilical vein

105. The fetal circulation is designed to:
   a) Maximize oxygen delivery to the lungs
   b) Minimize oxygen delivery to the liver
   c) Maximize oxygen delivery to the brain and heart
   d) Minimize oxygen delivery to the placenta

106. Which vessel carries deoxygenated blood from the fetus to the placenta?
   a) Umbilical artery
   b) Umbilical vein
   c) Ductus arteriosus
   d) Ductus venosus

107. What is the primary source of oxygen for the fetus?
   a) Fetal lungs
   b) Fetal liver
   c) Placenta
   d) Inferior vena cava

108. Which structure allows blood to flow directly from the right atrium to the left atrium in the fetus?
   a) Foramen ovale
   b) Ductus arteriosus
   c) Ductus venosus
   d) Umbilical vein

109. What happens to the foramen ovale after birth?
   a) It becomes the ligamentum arteriosum
   b) It remains open
   c) It becomes the fossa ovalis
   d) It becomes the umbilical ligament

110. Which of the following is NOT a feature of fetal circulation?
   a) High pulmonary vascular resistance
   b) Low systemic vascular resistance
   c) Presence of shunts
   d) High oxygen saturation in the umbilical arteries

Answer Key

1	c	2	b	3	b	4	b	5	a	6	c	7	b
8	c	9	a	10	c	11	c	12	a	13	c	14	a
15	c	16	b	17	a	18	b	19	b	20	b	21	c
22	a	23	b	24	c	25	b	26	b	27	b	28	b
29	c	30	a	31	a	32	b	33	a	34	b	35	b
36	b	37	a	38	c	39	b	40	b	41	d	42	b
43	c	44	a	45	b	46	c	47	c	48	a	49	c
50	a	51	a	52	a	53	c	54	b	55	c	56	b
57	c	58	a	59	c	60	a	61	c	62	d	63	c
64	b	65	a	66	c	67	b	68	a	69	b	70	b
71	b	72	b	73	c	74	a	75	c	76	c	77	c
78	b	79	a	80	a	81	a	82	b	83	a	84	a
85	c	86	a	87	c	88	a	89	c	90	d	91	b
92	b	93	b	94	b	95	b	96	c	97	b	98	a
99	c	100	b	101	a	102	b	103	a	104	a	105	c
106	a	107	c	108	a	109	c	110	d				

14

Development of Haematopoiesis and Blood Vascular System

K. Archana[1], M.P.S. Tomar[1], Ratnesh Kr. Choudhary[2] and Dangeti V.V.N.D. Prasad[3]

[1]*Department of Veterinary Anatomy Sri Venkateswara Veterinary University, Tirupati*
[2]*Department of Veterinary Anatomy, BVC, Bihar Animal Sciences University, Patna, Bihar*
[3]*Section of Veterinary Anatomy, ICAR-IVRI, Izatnagar, Bareilly, Uttar Pradesh*

Introduction

Cardiovascular system consists of heart and blood vessels which include both arteries and veins. The formation of blood vessels occurs in two stages-vasculogenesis and angiogenesis. Blood islands are formed on the yolk sac by clusters of mesodermal cells. Vasculogenesis i.e., formation of blood vessels starts during third week of gestation in the blood islands. It starts first in the yolk sac and later in the allantois. Angiogenesis describes budding and sprouting of new vessels from the existing vessels. The adult heart is a modified blood vessel. The cardiogenic plate lies ventral to the pericardial coelom in the third week gestation. The position gets reversed with the forward growth of the head and folding of the embryo. Two endocardial tubes appear by the end of 6 to 7 somite stage which fuse to form the primitive heart in the 8 to 9 somite stage. The parts of the endocardial tube are- sinus venosus, atrium, ventricle, bulbus cordis and truncus arteriosus. The four chambered heart is formed by the formation of endocardial cushions, interatrial septum, interventricular septum and spiral septum. The interatrial septum includes the formation of septum primum and septum secundum.

Oxygenated blood from the placenta enters the embryo by a large umbilical vein which enters the liver of the developing embryo. It is conveyed to the posterior vena cava through ductus venosus. The blood from the vena cava enters the right atrium which is sent to the left atrium through foramen ovale. Blood then enters the left ventricle and transmitted to all the parts through the aorta), The umbilical arteries arising from the aorta transport blood to placenta for oxygenation. After birth, lungs become functional as the placental circulation ceases.

The formation of arterial system involves the modification of aortic arches, ventral aorta, dorsal aorta and its dorsal, ventral and lateral branches. Aortic arches appear sequentially and connect cranial portions of dorsal aorta with ventral aorta)The venous system is derived from the remnants of the cardinal system and vitelline veins and to a lesser extent the umbilical veins.

Prenatal haematopoeisis in vertebrates occurs in two successive stages and in two different anatomical sites. A transient extraembryonic phase in the yolk sac is followed by a definitive intra embryonic phase at the viscinity of the dorsal aorta referred to as aorta-gonad- mesonephros (AGM). The activity extends from the yolk sac to liver,spleen and finally to bone marrow as embryogenesis proceeds. Toward the end of foetal life spleen is primarily an erythropoietic organ which aids in transfer of haematopoeisis from foetal liver to the bone marrow.

Multiple Choice Questions

1. The cardiovascular system consists of
   a) Heart b) Arteries
   c) Veins d) All
2. Blood vessels formation occurs in these stages
   a) Vasculogenesis b) Angiogenesis
   c) Both d) Three stages
3. Blood islands are clusters of cells which are first formed in
   a) Yolk sac b) Allantois
   c) Chorion d) Amnion
4. Blood islands of Pander in domestic animals commence during
   a) First week of gestation b) Third week of gestation
   c) Fourth week of gestation d) Second week of gestation
5. Budding and sprouting of new vessels from existing vessels is called
   a) Vasculogenesis b) Angiogenesis
   c) Both d) None
6. The cardiogenic plate in the third week of gestation in animals is located
   a) Ventral to pericardial coelom b) Dorsal to pericardial coelom
   c) Lateral to pericardial coelom d) Not specific
7. The number of endocardial tubes in the 6 to 7 somite's stage
   a) One b) Two
   c) Three d) Four
8. The number of endocardial tubes in the 8 to 9 somite's stage
   a) One b) Two
   c) Three d) Four
9. The endothelial lining of the endothelial tubes in primitive heart give rise to
   a) Pericardium b) Epicardium
   c) Endocardium d) None of the above
10. The cardiac tube is anchored in the pericardial cavity initially by
    a) Dorsal mesocardium b) Ventral mesocardium
    c) Lateral mesocardium d) Both A and B

11. The endocardial cushions separate
    a) Atrioventricular ostium
    b) Interatrial septum
    c) Interventricular septum
    d) None of the above
12. The interatrial septum is formed by
    a) Septum primum
    b) Septum secundum
    c) Both A and B
    d) None of the above
13. The truncus arteriosus is divided by
    a) Septum primum
    b) Septum secundum
    c) Spiral septum
    d) Endocardial cushions
14. The Foramen ovale is formed by the
    a) Septum primum
    b) Septum secundum
    c) Spiral septum
    d) Endocardial cushions
15. Valve of the Foramen ovale is formed by
    a) Septum primum
    b) Septum secundum
    c) Spiral septum
    d) Endocardial cushions
16. The aortic trunk becomes continuous with
    a) Fourth aortic arches
    b) Sixth aortic arches
    c) Third aortic arches
    d) Second aortic arch
17. The pulmonary artery becomes continuous with
    a) Fourth aortic arches
    b) Sixth aortic arches
    c) Third aortic arches
    d) Second aortic arches
18. The number of horns in sinus venosus
    a) One
    b) Two
    c) Three
    d) Four
19. Oxygenated blood from the placenta enters embryo through
    a) Umbilical vein
    b) Umbilical artery
    c) Pulmonary artery
    d) Pulmonary vein
20. Oxygenated blood from the placenta is conveyed first to
    a) Spleen
    b) Liver
    c) Aorta
    d) Lungs
21. Oxygenated blood from the liver is conveyed to
    a) Posterior vena cava
    b) Anterior vena cava
    c) Kidney
    d) Lungs
22. Oxygenated blood from the liver is conveyed to Posterior vena cava by
    a) Ductus venosus
    b) Hepatic veins
    c) Anterior vena cava
    d) Both A and B
23. Blood from the pulmonary artery in foetus is sent to aorta through
    a) Ductus venosus
    b) Ductus arteriosus
    c) Anterior vena cava
    d) Both A and B

24. In the foetus blood passes from left to the right atrium through
    a) Foramen ovale b) Sinus venosus
    c) Spiral septum d) None
25. Blood from the foetus is returned to placenta through
    a) Umbilical arteries b) Umbilical vein
    c) Ductus venosus d) Ductus arteriosus
26. After birth, umbilical arteries are transformed into
    a) Fossa ovalis b) Ligamentum teres of liver
    c) Round ligaments of bladder d) Ligamentum venosus of liver
27. After birth, Foramen ovale is transformed into
    a) Fossa ovalis b) Ligamentum teres of liver
    c) Round ligaments of bladder d) Ligamentum venosus of liver
28. After birth, left umbilical vein is transformed into
    a) Fossa ovalis b) Ligamentum teres of liver
    c) Round ligaments of bladder d) Ligamentum venosus of liver
29. After birth, Ductus venosus is transformed into
    a) Fossa ovalis b) Ligamentum teres of liver
    c) Round ligaments of bladder d) Ligamentum venosus of liver
30. After birth, Ductus arteriosus is transformed into
    a) Ligamentum arteriosum b) Ligamentum teres of liver
    c) Round ligaments of bladder d) Ligamentum venosus of liver
31. The aortic arches connect
    a) Cranial portion of dorsal aorta with ventral aorta
    b) Caudal portion of dorsal aorta with ventral aorta
    c) Lateral portion of dorsal aorta with ventral aorta
    d) None of the above
32. The aortic arches pass through the mesenchyme of
    a) Foregut b) Branchial arches
    c) Hindgut d) Midgut
33. The truncus arteriosus is divided into
    a) Carotid and aorta
    b) Pulmonary trunk and carotid artery
    c) Dorsal Aorta and pulmonary trunk
    d) No division
34. The aortic sac is located between
    a) Ventral aorta and aortic arches
    b) Pulmonary trunk and carotid artery
    c) Dorsal Aorta and pulmonary trunk
    d) No division

35. The dorsal aortae in branchial area extend into the head as
    a) Ventral aorta and aortic arches
    b) Internal carotid arteries
    c) Dorsal Aorta and pulmonary trunk
    d) They do not extend into the head
36. The external carotid arteries are formed as outgrowths of the
    a) First aortic arches b) Second aortic arches
    c) Fourth aortic arches d) Third aortic arches
37. The common carotid arteries are extensions of
    a) First aortic arches b) Second aortic arches
    c) Fourth aortic arches d) Third aortic arches
38. The right brachial artery is formed by
    a) First aortic arches b) Right dorsal aorta
    c) Fourth aortic arches d) Both B and C
39. The aortic arch is formed by the left side of
    a) Aortic sac b) left dorsal aorta
    c) Fourth aortic arches d) All the above
40. The proximal part of pulmonary artery is formed by
    a) Sixth aortic arches b) Second aortic arches
    c) Fourth aortic arches d) Third aortic arches
41. The initial position of the heart in embryo
    a) Thorax b) Pharynx
    c) Abdomen d) Lumbar
42. The brachiocephalic trunk develops from
    a) Metanephric blastema b) Ureteric bud
    c) Aortic arch d) None
43. The major derivatives of the dorsal intersegmental branches of the aorta are
    a) Intercostal arteries b) Lumbar arteries
    c) Both A and B d) None
44. The left brachial artery in pigs arises from
    a) Aortic arch b) Brachiocephalic trunk
    c) portal vein d) Carotid artery
45. The left brachial artery in dogs arises from
    a) Brachiocephalic trunk b) Aortic arch
    c) portal vein d) Carotid artery
46. The left brachial in horse arises from
    a) Carotid artery b) Aortic arch
    c) Portal vein d) Brachiocephalic trunk

47. The left brachial in ox arises from
    a) Carotid artery b) Aortic arch
    c) Portal vein d) Brachiocephalic trunk
48. The adult venous system is derived from the remnants of
    a) Cardinal system b) Vitelline veins
    c) Both A and B d) None
49. The hepatic sinusoids are formed from
    a) Vitelline veins b) Septum transversum
    c) Portal veins d) All the above
50. The portal veins are formed from
    a) Vitelline veins b) Septum transversum
    c) Portal veins d) All the above
51. The venous systems opening into sinus venosus in foetus
    a) Umbilical veins b) Vitelline veins
    c) Cardinal veins d) All the above
52. The internal and external jugular veins arise from
    a) Cranial cardinal veins b) Caudal cardinal veins
    c) Vitelline veins d) Vena cava
53. The brachial veins arise from
    a) Caudal cardinal veins b) Cranial cardinal veins
    c) Vitelline veins d) Vena cava
54. The cranial vena cava arises from
    a) Caudal cardinal veins b) Vitelline veins
    c) Cranial cardinal veins d) Vena cava
55. The dorsal sinus arises from
    a) Caudal cardinal veins b) Vitelline veins
    c) Cranial cardinal veins d) Vena cava
56. The cerebral veins arise from
    a) Caudal cardinal veins b) Vitelline veins
    c) Cranial cardinal veins d) Vena cava
57. The mesonephros in the foetus is drained by
    a) Subcardinal veins b) Vitelline veins
    c) Portal veins d) Vena cava
58. Renal veins are derived from
    a) Portal veins b) Vitelline veins
    c) Right Subcardinal veins d) Vena cava
59. Testicular veins are derived from
    a) Portal veins b) Right Subcardinal veins
    c) Vitelline veins d) Vena cava

60. Ovarian veins are derived from
    a) Right Subcardinal veins
    b) Portal veins
    c) Vitelline veins
    d) Vena cava

61. The azygos vein on the right-side drains into
    a) Cranial vena cava
    b) Caudal vena cava
    c) Coronary sinus
    d) None

62. The azygos vein on the left side drains into
    a) Cranial vena cava
    b) Caudal vena cava
    c) Coronary sinus
    d) None

63. The azygos vein in formed by
    a) Cranial portion of caudal cardinal veins
    b) Cranial part of supracardinal veins
    c) Both unite to form
    d) None

64. Cardinal system is composed of
    a) Cranial and caudal veins
    b) Common cardinal veins
    c) Supra and subcardinal veins
    d) All the above

65. Four chambered heart is the result of formation of
    a) Interatrial septum
    b) Interventricular septum
    c) Both
    d) Spiral septum

66. The extraembryonic phase of haematopoiesis occurs in
    a) Yolk sac
    b) Liver
    c) Spleen
    d) Bone marrow

67. The intraembryonic phase of haematopoiesis occurs in
    a) Liver
    b) Spleen
    c) Bone marrow
    d) All

68. Prenatal haematopoiesis involves yolk sac from
    a) 4th week
    b) 5th week
    c) 6th week
    d) 8th to 16th week

69. Prenatal haematopoiesis involves body mesenchyme and blood vessels from
    a) 4th week
    b) 5th week
    c) 6th week
    d) 8th to 16th week

70. Prenatal haematopoiesis involves liver from
    a) 4th week
    b) 5th week
    c) 6th week
    d) 8th to 16th week

71. Prenatal haematopoiesis involves spleen from
    a) 4th week
    b) 5th week
    c) 6th week
    d) 8th to 16th week

72. Prenatal haematopoiesis involves thymus from
   a) 4th week   b) 5th week
   c) 8th to 16th week   d) 6th week
73. Prenatal haematopoiesis involves bone marrow from
   a) 4th week   b) 5th week
   c) 6th week   d) 16th week
74. Blood cell formation does not involve hepatic stage in
   a) Cow   b) dog
   c) fowl   d) horse
75. Non haematopoietic supporting cells are called
   a) Stromal cells   b) Stem cells
   c) Gonadal cells   d) None
76. Non haematopoietic support cells are
   a) Endothelial cells   b) Fibroblasts
   c) Cells of monocyte-macrophage series   d) All the above
77. Haematopoietic cells capable of giving rise to all cell lineages is present throughout lifetime of individual in
   a) Bone marrow   b) Spleen
   c) Thymus   d) None
78. Progenitor cells of blood cells arise from
   a) Stem cells   b) Committed stem cells
   c) Stromal Cells   d) marker cells
79. Progenitor cells are capable of differentiating into
   a) Myeloid lineage   b) Lymphoid lineage
   c) Both A and B   d) None
80. The number of stages in which haematopoiesis occurs in vertebrates
   a) Two   b) Three
   c) Four   d) Five
81. AGM during haematopoiesis means
   a) Anti -Gonad-Mesonephros   b) Aorta -Gonad-Mesonephros
   c) Artery -Gonad-Mesonephros   d) Aorta -Gamete-Mesonephros
82. Blood islands are formed by
   a) Extra embryonic mesodermal cells   b) Endoderm
   c) Ectoderm.   d) Both A and b.
83. The outer cells of the blood islands differentiate into
   a) Endothelial cells   b) Erythroblasts
   c) Lymphoblasts   d) None
84. The inner cells of the blood islands differentiate into
   a) Endothelial cells   b) Erythroblasts
   c) Lymphoblasts   d) None

85. The process of attraction of HSC (Haemopoietic stem cells) to bone marrow is termed
   a) Homing b) Pulling
   c) Levelling d) None
86. Committed cell lineage in formation of erythrocyte involves
   a) Erythrocyte CFU b) Proerythroblast
   c) Reticulocyte d) All
87. Committed cell lineage in formation of basophil involves
   a) Basophil CFU b) Myeloblast
   c) Basophilic myelocyte d) All
88. Committed cell lineage in formation of eosinophil involves
   a) Eosinophilic CFU b) Myeloblast
   c) Eosinophilic myelocyte d) All
89. Committed cell lineage in formation of mast cell involves
   a) Mast cell CFU b) Immature mast cell
   c) Both A and B d) Myeloblast
90. Committed cell lineage in formation of neutrophil involves
   a) Granulocyte macrophage CFU b) Myeloblast
   c) Neutrophilic myelocyte d) All
91. Committed cell lineage in formation of monocyte involves
   a) Granulocyte macrophage CFU b) Monoblast
   c) Promonocyte d) All
92. Committed cell lineage in formation of B-cell involves
   a) B lymphoid progenitor b) Pre-B-Cell
   c) Immature B cell d) All
93. Committed cell lineage in formation of T-cell involves
   a) T lymphoid precursor b) Pre-T-Cell
   c) Immature T cell d) All
94. The autosomal recessive disease involving haematopoietic system is
   a) Chediak Hagashi syndrome b) Leucocyte adhesion deficiency
   c) Wiskott Aldrich syndrome d) All
95. Gray collie syndrome is seen in
   a) Dogs b) Horses
   c) Monkeys d) Cattle
96. Gray collie syndrome affects
   a) Leucocytes b) Erythrocytes
   c) Both A and B d) Monocytes
97. What is the primary cause of inherited blood disorders in domestic animals
   a) Inherited enzymatic deficiencies b) Hemopoietic diseases
   c) Vascular system anomalies d) Immunodeficiency diseases

98. Which breed of dog is associated with inherited neutropenia

a) German Shepherd b) Golden Retriever

c) Gray Collie d) Labrador Retriever

99. What is the likely explanation for the embryogenesis of the hemopoietic part of the gray collie syndrome

a) Failure of seeding of the bone marrow by stem cells

b) Overproduction of stem cells

c) Defect in the vascular system

d) Immunodeficiency disease

100. What is the primary defect in combined immunodeficiency disease in Arabian foals

a) Failure of seeding of lymphatic organs with T- and B-lymphocytes

b) Defect in the vascular system

c) Overproduction of stem cells

d) Immunodeficiency disease

101. Which of the following is NOT a likely cause of inherited blood disorders in domestic animals

a) Inherited enzymatic deficiencies b) Hemopoietic diseases

c) Vascular system anomalies d) Trauma

102. What is the primary source of the adult venous system

a) Cardinal system b) Vitelline veins

c) Umbilical veins d) All of the above

103. What is the fate of the right umbilical vein during embryonic development

a) It enlarges and becomes a major vein b) It disappears

c) It remains unchanged d) It becomes a lymphatic vessel

104. What is the ductus venosus

a) A channel connecting the left umbilical vein to the sinus venosus

b) A channel connecting the left umbilical vein to the right vitelline vein

c) A channel connecting the right umbilical vein to the sinus venosus

d) A channel connecting the right umbilical vein to the left vitelline vein

105. What is the fate of the left umbilical vein during embryonic development?

a) It enlarges and becomes a major vein b) It disappears

c) It remains unchanged d) It becomes a lymphatic vessel

106. What is the portal vein derived from

a) Left vitelline vein

b) Right vitelline vein

c) Middle anastomosis of the vitelline veins

d) All of the above

107. What is the function of the hepatic sinusoids during embryonic development
   a) To filter the blood
   b) To store the blood
   c) To serve as an "overflow" area for the heart
   d) To produce blood cells

108. What is the fate of the cranial portion of the left vitelline vein during embryonic development
   a) It disappears
   b) It remains unchanged
   c) It becomes the left subclavian vein
   d) It becomes part of the portal vein

109. What is the result of the formation of the ductus venosus
   a) The left umbilical vein becomes smaller
   b) The left umbilical vein becomes larger
   c) The right umbilical vein becomes larger
   d) The right umbilical vein becomes smaller

110. What is the fate of the right vitelline vein during embryonic development
   a) It disappears
   b) It remains unchanged
   c) It becomes part of the portal vein
   d) It becomes the inferior vena cava

111. What is the result of the rotation of the stomach to the left during embryonic development
   a) The left vitelline vein becomes smaller
   b) The left vitelline vein becomes larger
   c) The right vitelline vein becomes smaller
   d) The right vitelline vein becomes larger

Answer Key

1	a	2	c	3	a	4	b	5	b	6	a	7	b
8	a	9	c	10	d	11	a	12	c	13	c	14	b
15	a	16	a	17	b	18	b	19	a	20	b	21	a
22	d	23	b	24	a	25	a	26	c	27	a	28	b
29	d	30	a	31	a	32	b	33	c	34	a	35	b
36	d	37	d	38	d	39	d	40	a	41	b	42	c
43	c	44	a	45	b	46	d	47	d	48	c	49	a
50	a	51	d	52	a	53	b	54	c	55	c	56	c
57	a	58	c	59	b	60	a	61	a	62	c	63	c
64	d	65	c	66	a	67	d	68	a	69	b	70	c

71	d	72	c	73	d	74	c	75	a	76	d	77	a
78	b	79	c	80	a	81	b	82	d	83	a	84	b
85	a	86	d	87	d	88	d	89	c	90	d	91	d
92	d	93	d	94	a	95	a	96	a	97	a	98	c
99	a	100	a	101	d	102	d	103	b	104	b	105	a
106	d	107	c	108	a	109	b	110	c	111	b		

15

Development of Nervous System

Ayesha Boddupalli

Department of Veterinary Anatomy, SOA, Bhubaneshwar, Odisha

Introduction

The nervous system is an intricate network that plays a crucial role in coordinating and regulating bodily functions, allowing organisms to interact with their environment. This complex system is fundamental for the existence, enabling to sense the world, process information, and respond to stimuli. Comprised of billions of specialized cells called neurons. The nervous system is responsible for various functions, from reflex actions to complex thought processes. The nervous system is a highly organized and complex network that serves as the primary means of communication within the body of all animals, including domesticated species. Understanding the anatomy and function of the nervous system is critical in veterinary medicine, as it governs essential processes such as locomotion, sensation, cognition, and homeostasis. Comprising the central nervous system (CNS) and peripheral nervous system (PNS), the nervous system enables the coordination of reflexes and voluntary movements, facilitating interactions with the environment.

Structural Organization: the CNS is composed of the brain and spinal cord, which are protected by the bony encasement of the skull and vertebral column, respectively. The brain varies significantly across species, reflecting adaptations to specific ecological niches and behaviors. For instance, the canine brain shows notable development in areas associated with olfaction, whereas the equine brain has adaptations for vision and balance, crucial for flight responses. The spinal cord serves as a conduit for neural signals between the brain and the peripheral nerves. It is organized segmentally, with spinal nerves emerging from specific regions. This segmentation corresponds to the vertebral column and is vital for diagnosing spinal cord injuries and diseases in animals. Each spinal nerve innervates specific muscle groups and areas of the skin, forming a somatic map essential for clinical examination and treatment.

Neurons and Neuroglia: Neurons are the functional units of the nervous system, specialized for the transmission of electrochemical signals. In veterinary anatomy, it is essential to understand the structure of neurons, which includes the cell body, dendrites, and axon. Neurons can be classified into various types—sensory (afferent), motor (efferent), and interneurons—each playing distinct roles in reflex arcs and neural circuits. Neuroglia, or glial cells, provide support, nourishment, and protection for neurons. In veterinary practice, the role of glial cells in pathology is increasingly recognized, particularly in conditions such as neuroinflammation and neurodegeneration. For example, astrocytes play a crucial role in maintaining the blood-brain barrier, and their dysfunction can lead to significant neurological disorders in animals.

Functional Divisions: The nervous system is functionally divided into the somatic and autonomic nervous systems. The somatic nervous system controls voluntary muscle movements and sensory information from the periphery to the CNS. This system is particularly relevant in veterinary anatomy for understanding reflexes and motor control in animals, such as the withdrawal reflex, which protects against injury. The autonomic nervous system (ANS) regulates involuntary physiological functions, including heart rate, digestion, and respiratory rate. It is further divided into the sympathetic and parasympathetic systems, which often have opposing effects. In veterinary medicine, understanding the ANS is crucial for managing stress responses in animals, particularly during surgery or stressful situations. For instance, sympathetic activation prepares the body for "fight or flight" responses, while parasympathetic activation promotes rest and digestion.

Sensory Pathways and Motor Control: Sensory pathways are integral to the nervous system, allowing animals to perceive their environment. Different sensory modalities, such as vision, hearing, smell, taste, and touch, are processed through specific neural pathways. In veterinary anatomy, the assessment of sensory function is vital for diagnosing neurological conditions. For example, testing a dog's ability to hear can indicate potential inner ear issues or neurological dysfunction. Motor control involves complex interactions between the CNS and muscles. The motor cortex, located in the forebrain, plays a pivotal role in planning and executing voluntary movements. The brainstem and spinal cord are also critical for coordinating reflexive movements. Understanding these pathways is essential for veterinary practitioners when diagnosing conditions that affect mobility, such as degenerative myelopathy in dogs or equine laryngeal paralysis.

Neurotransmission and Communication: Neurotransmitters are biochemical messengers that facilitate communication between neurons at synapses. Different neurotransmitters, such as acetylcholine, dopamine, and serotonin, play various roles in modulating mood, motor control, and cognitive function. In veterinary practice, knowledge of neurotransmitter systems is important for understanding behaviors and developing treatments for conditions like anxiety or aggression in pets.

Clinical Relevance: A thorough understanding of the nervous system is paramount in diagnosing and treating neurological disorders in animals. Conditions such as seizures, spinal cord injuries, and neurodegenerative diseases can significantly impact an animal's quality of life. Veterinary neurologists rely on advanced imaging techniques, such as MRI and CT scans, to assess structural abnormalities within the CNS. Moreover, recognizing the signs of neurological dysfunction—such as altered behavior, weakness, or ataxia—is crucial for early intervention and effective management. Veterinary practitioners must be well-versed in the anatomy and function of the nervous system to provide comprehensive care, including surgical interventions for conditions like intervertebral disc disease in dogs or traumatic brain injuries in cats.

Conclusion: the nervous system is a vital component of veterinary anatomy, influencing all aspects of an animal's health and behavior. Its intricate structure and multifaceted functions underscore the importance of understanding neuroanatomy in veterinary medicine. From sensory processing to motor control and neurochemical communication, the nervous system enables animals to adapt to their environment, maintain homeostasis, and respond to challenges. As research continues to advance our knowledge of the nervous system, veterinarians will be better equipped to diagnose and treat a range of neurological conditions, ultimately improving the welfare of the animals in their care.

Multiple Choice Questions

1. Dura mater develops from
   a) Ectoderm b) Mesoderm
   c) Endoderm d) All of these
2. Pia mater is derived from
   a) Neural crest b) Endoderm
   c) Mesoderm d) Ectoderm
3. Arachnoid mater is derived from
   a) Neural crest b) Endoderm
   c) Mesoderm d) Ectoderm
4. Neural crest cells are derived from
   a) Ectoderm b) Endoderm
   c) Mesoderm d) Both b & c
5. The 6th pharyngeal arch and its derivatives are mostly innervated by nerve.
   a) Facial b) Trigeminal
   c) Glossopharyngeal d) Recurrent laryngeal
6. The 3rd brachial arch and its derivatives are innervated by nerve.
   a) Facial b) Trigeminal
   c) Glossopharyngeal d) Vagus
7. The 1" pharyngeal arch and its derivatives are mostly innervated by nerve.
   a) Facial b) Trigeminal
   c) Glossopharyngeal d) Vagus
8. The 2nd pharyngeal arch and its derivatives are innervated by nerve.
   a) Facial b) Trigeminal
   c) Glossopharyngeal d) Vagus
9. Neural crest cells gives rise to cells.
   a) Parafollicular b) Melanocyte and chromaffin
   c) Odontoblast d) All of these
10. Spongioblasts differentiate into neuroglia cells like
    a) Astrocytes b) Microglia
    c) Oligodendrocytes d) both a & c
11. Spongioblasts of the neural tube are originates from .
    a) Ectoderm b) Mesoderm
    c) Endoderm d) Both a & c
12. Microgliocytes of the CNS originate from .
    a) Ectoderm b) Mesoderm
    c) Endoderm d) Both a & c

13. Number of layers are present in embryonic neural tube.
    a) 5 b) 3
    c) 2 d) 4
14. The layers of the embryonic neural tube are named as .
    a) Marginal b) Germinal
    c) Mantle d) All of these
15. Are called as the ad-luminal layer of the embryonic neural tube.
    a) Marginal b) Germinal
    c) Ventricular d) Both b & c
16. is the mid-layer of the embryonic neural tube.
    a) Marginal b) Mantle
    c) Ventricular d) Germinal
17. The outer-layer of the embryonic neural tube is the layer.
    a) Marginal b) Mantle
    c) Ventricular d) Germinal
18. The layer of the embryonic neural tube is the area of active cell division.
    a) Marginal b) Mantle
    c) Germinal d) Ventricular
19. The Germinal layer of the embryonic neural tube carries.
    a) Cell bodies of neuroepithelial cells b) Presumptive glial cells
    c) Immature neurons d) All of these
20. Layer of neural tube carries axonal processes of developing neurons.
    a) Marginal b) Mantle
    c) Germinal d) All of these
21. The sulcus demarcates the dorsal alar plate and ventral basal plate of mantle of the developing spinal cord
    a) Dorso-median b) Ventro-median
    c) Limiting d) Coronary
22. The mantle layer of the developing spinal cord contains plate.
    a) Alar b) Basal
    c) Neural d) Both a & b
23. Function is seen in most of the alar plate-neurons of the developing spinal cord have.
    a) Motor b) Sensory
    c) Sustentacular d) Mixed
24. Function is seen in most of the basal plate-neurons of the developing spinal cord have functions.
    a) Motor b) Sensory
    c) Mixed d) Sustentacular

25. The gray matter of the spinal cord develops from its layer.
    a) Ventricular b) Mantle
    c) Marginal d) Both a & b
26. The white matter of the spinal cord develops from its layer.
    a) Ventricular b) Marginal
    c) Mantle d) Medullary
27. The ependymal cell layer of spinal cord develops from layer.
    a) Ventricular b) Marginal
    c) Mantle d) Cortical
28. The ganglia develop from .
    a) Endoderm b) Mesoderm
    c) Sclerotome d) Ectoderm
29. Zone forms the neurons, neurglial cells and germinal cells.
    a) Ependymal b) Mantle zone
    c) Marginal zone d) All of the above
30. Zone consists of neuroblasts and spongioblasts.
    a) Ependymal b) Mantle zone
    c) Marginal zone d) All of the above
31. The cytoplasmic processes that extends laterally from neuroblasts of mantle layer forms zone.
    a) Ependymal b) Mantle zone
    c) Marginal zone d) All of the above

Answer Key

1	b	2	a	3	a	4	a	5		6		7	
8	b	9	d	10	d	11	b	12	b	13	b	14	d
15	d	16	b	17	a	18	c	19	d	20	a	21	c
22	d	23	b	24	a	25	b	26	b	27	a	28	d
29	a	30	b	31	c								

16

Development of Musculo-Skeletal System

Ratnesh Kumar Choudhary[1], Nidhi Gupta[2] and Tanmoy Rana

[1]Department of Veterinary Anatomy, BVC, BASU, Patna, Bihar

[2]Department of Veterinary Anatomy, College of Veterinary Sciences and Animal Husbandry, Jabalpur, Madhya Pradesh

[3]Department of Veterinary Clinical compelx, West Bengal University of Animal & Fishery Sciences, Kolkata, West Bengal

Introduction

- Overview of the development of the musculoskeletal system, including bones, cartilage, joints, and muscle types within skeletal and cardiac systems.

Development of the Musculoskeletal System

Mesoderm Contributions

- **Mesodermal Derivatives**
  - Gives rise to skeletal muscle, skin dermis, endochondral bones, and joints.
- **Notochord and Somite Formation**
  - The notochord induces the paraxial mesoderm to form somites, with somitomeres developing rostrally to the notochord in the head)
- **Somite Differentiation**
  - Each somite differentiates into three regions:
    - **Sclerotome (medial)**: Forms most of the axial skeleton (vertebrae, ribs, base of the skull).
    - **Dermatome (lateral)**: Migrates to form the dermis of the skin.
    - **Myotome (middle)**: Migrates to form skeletal muscles. Individual adult muscles arise from the merger of adjacent myotomes.

Muscle Development

- **Origins of Muscle Tissue**:
  - All skeletal muscle derives from paraxial mesoderm forming somites and somitomeres, with the exception of iris musculature (derived from optic cup ectoderm).
  - Cardiac and smooth muscles originate from splanchnic mesoderm.

- **Myotome Differentiation**
  - Myotome cells differentiate into myoblasts, which fuse to form multinucleate myocytes (muscle fibers).
  - Myocytes synthesize myosin and actin, aligning to produce striated muscle appearance.
- **Muscle Growth and Regeneration**:
  - Each anatomical muscle is genetically allocated a specific number of myoblasts determined by birth; postnatally, growth occurs via hypertrophy, as hyperplasia (regeneration) of adult muscle cells does not occur.
- **Innervation and Muscle Grouping**
  - Adjacent myotomes merge to form broad muscles that are segmentally innervate d) Myotome accumulations segregate into:
  - **Dorsal mass (epimere)**: Innervated by dorsal branches of spinal nerves (epaxial muscles).
  - **Ventral mass (hypomere)**: Innervated by ventral branches of spinal nerves (hypaxial muscles).

Bone Development

- **Types of Bone Formation**
  - Most bones are formed endochondrally (ossification of cartilage precursor).
  - Bones of the calvaria and face form intramembranously (osteoblasts arise from ectomesenchyme, not chondroblasts).
- **Embryological Origins of the Skeleton**
  - **Paraxial mesoderm**: Forms sclerotomes that give rise endochondrally to the axial skeleton.
  - **Somatic mesoderm**: Forms endochondral appendicular bones.
  - **Ectomesenchyme (neural crest)**: Forms intramembranous bones of the calvaria and face.

Endochondral Bone Formation

- Local mesenchyme condenses, differentiating into chondroblasts that secrete a matrix forming a cartilage model surrounded by perichondral fibrous tissue. Ossification occurs first in the diaphysis (primary ossification), followed by the epiphyses (secondary ossification).

Axial Skeleton

- **Formation of Vertebrae and Ribs**
  - Sclerotomes give rise to vertebrae and ribs.
  - The sternum develops from local somatic mesenchyme through chondrification and ossification.
  - Intervertebral discs form from sclerotome mesenchyme and notochord)
- **Rib Development**
  - Ribs develop as extensions of thoracic vertebrae processes.

Appendicular Skeleton

- Bone, cartilage, and connective tissue of the limbs arise from local somatic mesoderm of the limb bud, condensing to form cartilage models of limb bones.

Skull Development

- **Base of Cranium**
  - Develops endochondrally from sclerotomes of somitomeres and the first four occipital somites.
- **Calvaria and Face**
  - Flat bones of the calvaria and face develop intramembranously from ectomesenchyme.
  - Intramembranous bones articulate via sutures, with widened areas called fontanels.
- **Mandible Development**
  - Has a complex origin involving both endochondral and intramembranous development.
- **Auditory Ossicles**
  - Arise endochondrally from pharyngeal arches I (malleus and incus) and II (stapes).

Joint Development

- Mesenchyme condensation creates an interzone region within perichondral tissue, connecting adjacent cartilage models.
- **Synovial Joint Formation**:
  - Cavitation occurs at the center of the interzone, with bordering tissue becoming the synovial membrane.
  - Perichondral tissue surrounding the interzone forms the joint capsule, with localized thickenings forming ligaments.

Multiple Choice Questions

1. Skeletal muscles develop from ----------germ layer

   a) Ectoderm b) Mesoderm

   c) Endoderm d) All of these

2. Somite develop from ------------------ part of mesoderm

   a) Paraxial mesoderm b) Intermediate mesoderm

   c) Lateral plate mesoderm d) All of these

3. In mammals------ pair of somitomeres develop

   a) 6 **b) 7**

   c) 8 d) 5

4. For development of one vertebra ---------- somites are needed

   a) One pair b) Two pair

   c) Three pair d) One somite

5. Signalling molecules from ------genes differentiate the medio-ventral region of somites to sclerotome
   a) Sonic hedgehog b) Wnt gene
   c) Muscle specific gene d) None of these
6. Paraxial mesoderm cranial to otic placodes divides into ---------
   a) Somite b) Somatomere
   c) Metamere d) All of these
7. Myotomes give rise to muscles of -----------region
   a) Trunk b) Neck
   c) Limb d) All of these
8. One skeletal muscle may be derived from
   a) One myotome b) More than one myotome
   c) Both a & B d) None of these
9. Epaxial muscles of body are developed from
   a) Epimeres b) Hypomeres
   c) Both a and b d) Sclerotome
10. Smooth muscles of the body derive from----
    a) Somatic mesoderm b) Splanchnic mesoderm
    c) Somatometres d) Myotome
11. Ciliary muscles of eye derive from
    a) Mesenchyme b) Somatic mesoderm
    c) Splanchnic mesoderm d) Neural crest cells
12. Myoblast are differentiated from myotomes by -------- factors
    a) Wnt b) Shh
    c) MyoD d) All of these
13. Fibrocartilage contains ------------type of collagen fibres
    a) Type II collagen b) Type I collagen
    c) Type III collagen d) All of these
14. The cartilaginous model in endochondral ossification is made up of
    a) Hyaline cartilage b) Elastic cartilage
    c) Fibrocartilage d) Mesenchyme
15. The length of bone increases by --------
    a) Appositional growth b) Interstitial growth
    c) Calcification d) None of these
16. Basal plate cartilage primordia give rise to -------
    a) Basilar occipital b) Lateral occipital
    c) Petrous temporal bone d) Both a and b
17. Meckel's cartilage of mandibular arch give rise to-----------
    a) Malleus and incus b) Malleus and stapes
    c) Incus and stapes d) Malleus, incus and stapes

18. Stapes of middle ear develop from----
    a) Meckel's cartilage
    b) Reichert's cartilage
    c) Otic capsule
    d) Both a and b
19. The primary centre of ossification is for------- in long bones
    a) Epiphysis
    b) Diaphysis
    c) Both a&b
    d) None of these
20. Cartilagenous neurocranium includes----
    a) Parachordal cartilage
    b) Hypophyseal cartilage
    c) Prechordal cartilage
    d) All of these
21. Fontanelles present in -----------region
    a) Skull
    b) Neck
    c) Trunk
    d) Limb
22. Vertebral column develop from--------structure on either side of neural tube
    a) Perichordal blastema/tube
    b) Notochord
    c) Somatomeres
    d) All of these
23. The cranial displacement of spinal cord is greater in ------region
    a) Cervical
    b) Lumbar
    c) Coccygeal
    d) Lumbar, sacral and coccygeal
24. First three occipital somites participate in formation of---------
    a) Cervical vertebrae
    b) Base of cranium
    c) Roof of cranium
    d) Sternum
25. Spina bifida condition occurs when there is -----------
    a) Fusion of two vertebra
    b) Failure in fusion of neural arches
    c) Failure of sclerotome differentiation
    d) All of these
26. Schistosomus reflexus includes ------- abnormalities
    a) cleft sternum
    b) dorsal reflexion of ribs
    c) fail to close body wall
    d) all of these
27. During evolution ------ digits are reduced in bovine
    a) absence of 1st digit
    b) 2 and 5 digits as non-weight bearing
    c) 3 and 4 digits as non-weight bearing
    d) Both a & b
28. Syndactyly is a consequence -----------
    a) Failure in breakdown of interdigital mesoderm
    b) Incomplete formation of digital rays
    c) Decondensation of mesenchyme
    d) All of these

29. The arrectores pilorum muscle of skin derived from ----------germ layer
    a) Ectoderm b) Mesoderm
    c) Endoderm d) Both a&b
30. ------------number of ossification centres are present in development of femur
    a) Four b) Five
    c) Two d) Three
31. Synovial joints are formed when mesenchymal cells between ends of developing bone ---
    a) Differentiate into fibrous CT
    b) Differentiate into hyaline cartilage
    c) Differentiate into fibrocartilage
    d) Central apoptosis and peripheral differentiation
32. Limb buds are developed from------
    a) Sclerotome b) Somatopleuric mesoderm
    c) Splanchnopleuric mesoderm d) All of these
33. ------------centre of ossification appears for each sternebra
    a) Two b) Three
    c) One d) Seven
34. Abnormal ventral curvature of vertebral column refers to---
    a) Kyphosis b) Lordosis
    c) Both a&b d) Scoliosis
35. Cardiac muscles develop from-----
    a) Sclerotome b) Somatopleuric mesoderm
    c) Splanchnopleuric mesoderm d) Myotome
36. Os-coxae develop from --------number of ossification centres
    a) One centre for each bone b) Two centre for each bone
    c) Total six centres d) Total eight centres
37. In arthrogryposis development of ----------- part is affected
    a) Vertebrae b) Joints of limbs
    c) Skull bones d) Ribs
38. Premature ossification of physis is termed as
    a) Hypochondroplasia b) Achondroplasia
    c) Hyperchondroplasia d) none of these
39. Phocomelia refers to-----
    a) Underdeveloped limbs b) Underdeveloped vertebrae
    c) Malformed trunk d) Presence of extra digit
40. First secreted component of osteoid is --------
    a) Reticular fibers b) Collagen fibers
    c) Elastic fibers d) Ground substance

41. Secondary centre of ossification are located in ---------------
    a) Diaphysis b) Epiphysis
    c) Both a &b d) None of these
42. During development limbs undergo a series of -------------
    a) Twisting b) Rotation
    c) Angular movement d) revolving movement
43. Fusion of two or more adjacent vertebrae is termed as------
    a) Spina bifida b) Block Vertebra
    c) Kyphosis d) Scoliosis
44. Achondroplastic animals has-------------------abnormalities
    a) Short limb extremities b) Enlarged heads
    c) Flattened face d) All of these
45. Second phalanx develop from -------------number of ossification centres
    a) Two b) Three
    c) One d) Four
46. Intercostal muscles of thorax develop from--------
    a) Mesenchyme b) Segmented hypomeres
    c) Fused hypomeres d) Epimeres
47. Cartilage gets its nutrition by------------
    a) Direct blood supply b) Process of diffusion
    c) both a & b d) Not require nutrition
48. Isogenous groups within lacunae have-------------- cells
    a) Osteocytes b) Chondroblasts
    c) Chondrocytes d) Fibroblast
49. Haversian system develop in --------------type of bone
    a) Cancellous bone b) Spongy bone
    c) Compact bone d) All of these
50. Bone remodelling occurs in -------------stages
    a) Throughout foetal life b) Throughout the life
    c) both a & b d) Not occur in normal development
51. The condition of abnormal dense bone with obliterated marrow cavity refers to
    a) Osteogenesis imperfecta b) Osteopetrosis
    c) Osteoporosis d) Osteomalacia
52. Which mesoderm is the precursor of the somites in the trunk and the somitomeres in the head)
    a) Paraxial mesoderm b) Intermediate mesoderm
    c) Lateral plate mesoderm d) All of these.
53. Striated muscle of the iris originate from
    a) Mesenchyme b) Somatic mesoderm
    c) Splanchnic mesoderm d) Neural crest ectoderm

54. Smooth muscle of the digestive and respiratory tracts arises from
  a) Somitomere 1 and 2 b) Somatic mesoderm
  c) Splanchnic mesoderm d) None of these
55. Smooth muscle of the blood vessels arises from
  a) Somitomere 1 and 2 b) Somatic mesoderm
  c) Splanchnic mesoderm d) None of these
56. Fast- contracting muscle fibers have
  a) One LC_1, two LC_2 and one LC_3 light chain subunits
  b) Two LC_1 and two LC_2 chain
  c) One LC_1 and one LC_2 chain
  d) None of the above
57. Slow- contracting muscle fibers contain
  a) One LC_1, two LC_2 and one LC_3 light chain subunits
  b) Two LC_1 and two LC_2 chain
  c) One LC_1 and one LC_2 chain
  d) None of the above
58. Muscle of the tongue and larynx arises from the
  a) Somitomere 1 and 2 b) Occipital somites
  c) Splanchnic mesoderm d) Trunk somites
59. Diaphragm derived from
  a) Somitomere 1 and 2 b) Occipital somites
  c) Splanchnic mesoderm d) Trunk somites
60. Cardiac muscle derived from
  a) Somitomere 1 and 2 b) Occipital somites
  c) Splanchnic mesoderm d) Trunk somites
61. The vertebral column and ribs, being derived from the-------------portion of the somites
  a) Sclerotomal b) Dermatomal
  c) Myotomal d) None of these
62. In birds the bones of the cranial vault are derived from
  a) Cephalic mesoderm b) Neural crest
  c) Splanchnic mesoderm d) Somatic mesoderm
63. The outer wall of the somite contributes to the formation of the connective tissue layer of the skin is called
  a) Myotome b) Dermatome
  c) Sclerotome d) None of these
64. The dorsal part of the inner wall of the somite is the source of somatic muscle is called
  a) Myotome b) Dermatome
  c) Sclerotome d) None of these

65. The cartilaginous capsules of the sense organs (nose, eye, ear) develop from
   a) Skeletogenic mesenchyme b) Somatopleuric mesoderm
   c) Splanchnic mesoderm d) None of these
66. In the horse, all digital blastema except the ------------are lost in the embryo
   a) First b) Second
   c) Third d) Fourth
67. The viscerocranium (Jaws and related bones) develops from
   a) Skeletogenic mesenchyme b) Ectomesenchyme
   c) Mesodermal mesenchyme d) None
68. The neurocranium (Brain case) develops from
   a) Skeletogenic mesenchyme b) Ectomesenchyme
   c) Mesodermal mesenchyme d) None
69. The --------------- skull is the high nuchal crest of the occipital bone.
   a) Porcine b) Caprine
   c) Carnivore d) Ruminant
70. Limb anomalies are the most common congenital musculoskeletal defects in
   a) Domestic animals b) Birds
   c) Wild animals d) Aquatic animals

Answer Key

1	b	2	a	3	b	4	a	5	a	6	a	7	b
8	c	9	a	10	b	11	d	12	d	13	b	14	a
15	b	16	d	17	a	18	b	19	b	20	d	21	a
22	a	23	d	24	b	25	b	26	d	27	d	28	a
29	a	30	a	31	c	32	b	33	c	34	b	35	c
36	a	37	b	38	b	39	a	40	b	41	b	42	b
43	b	44	d	45	b	46	b	47	b	48	c	49	c
50	c	51	b	52	a	53	d	54	c	55	b	56	a
57	b	58	b	59	d	60	c	61	a	62	b	63	b
64	a	65	a	66	c	67	b	68	c	69	a	70	a

17

Development of Digestive System

Ayesha Boddupalli

Department of Veterinary Anatomy, Siksha 'O' Anusandhan, Bhubaneshwar, Odisha

Introduction

Introduction: The digestive system, or gastrointestinal (GI) tract, plays a fundamental role in the overall health and well-being of animals. In veterinary anatomy, understanding the structure and function of the digestive system is essential for diagnosing and treating various disorders that affect food intake, digestion, and nutrient absorption. This complex system is responsible for the mechanical and chemical breakdown of food, the absorption of nutrients, and the elimination of waste, making it crucial for maintaining homeostasis in animal species.

Structural Organization: The digestive system can be divided into two main categories: the gastrointestinal tract and the accessory digestive organs. The gastrointestinal tract is a continuous tube extending from the mouth to the anus and includes the oral cavity, esophagus, stomach, small intestine, large intestine, rectum, and anus. Each segment of the GI tract is specialized for specific functions, reflecting the dietary habits and evolutionary adaptations of different species.

Mouth and Esophagus: The digestive process begins in the mouth, where food is mechanically broken down by teeth and mixed with saliva, which contains enzymes like amylase that initiate carbohydrate digestion. The esophagus serves as a conduit for food, transporting it to the stomach through peristaltic movements.

Stomach: The stomach is a muscular organ that serves as a site for food storage and initial digestion. It secretes gastric juices, including hydrochloric acid and pepsin, to denature proteins and activate digestive enzymes. The morphology of the stomach can vary significantly across species.

In ruminants—such as cattle, sheep, and goats—the stomach is uniquely adapted for processing fibrous plant material through a complex structure consisting of four compartments: the rumen, reticulum, omasum, and abomasum.

1. Rumen: The largest compartment, the rumen, acts as a fermentation chamber where microbial digestion occurs. It is lined with a stratified squamous epithelium and contains millions of microorganisms, including bacteria, protozoa, and fungi, that help break down cellulose and other complex carbohydrates. The rumen's large surface area, facilitated by papillae, enhances absorption of volatile fatty acids (VFAs) produced during fermentation, which serve as a primary energy source for ruminants.

2. Reticulum: The reticulum, often referred to as the "honeycomb" due to its internal structure, works closely with the rumen. It further aids in fermentation and acts as a sorting area for particles. The reticulum plays a crucial role in the regurgitation of food during rumination, allowing animals to re-chew and further break down their food, enhancing nutrient absorption.
3. Omasum: The omasum, characterized by its many folds, functions to absorb water and nutrients, including VFAs and electrolytes, from the digested material. The structure of the omasum increases its surface area, facilitating efficient absorption while also acting as a sieve to filter out larger particles that are not yet ready for digestion in the abomasum.
4. Abomasum: The abomasum is the true stomach of ruminants, functioning similarly to the monogastric stomach. It secretes gastric juices, including hydrochloric acid and digestive enzymes, to further break down proteins and prepare the contents for passage into the small intestine. The abomasum's enzymatic activity is critical for the digestion of microbial proteins produced in the rumen.

Small Intestine: Following the stomach, the small intestine is divided into three regions: the duodenum, jejunum, and ileum. This section is the primary site for nutrient absorption. The surface area of the small intestine is greatly increased by villi and microvilli, enhancing its absorptive capacity. Enzymatic digestion continues here, aided by pancreatic enzymes and bile from the liver, which emulsifies fats.

Large Intestine: The large intestine is responsible for the absorption of water and electrolytes, as well as the fermentation of indigestible food matter in some species. The colon and rectum store fecal material before its elimination. The structure of the large intestine can vary; for example, the equine large intestine is particularly large and adapted for the fermentation of cellulose.

Functional Anatomy: The functional anatomy of the digestive system is intricately linked to an animal's diet and feeding behaviors. Herbivores, carnivores, and omnivores exhibit distinct adaptations that reflect their nutritional requirements. Ruminants possess a specialized stomach structure that enables them to break down cellulose through microbial fermentation, illustrating a significant evolutionary adaptation. In contrast, carnivorous animals, such as cats and dogs, have shorter digestive tracts and a more acidic gastric environment, allowing for rapid digestion and absorption of proteins and fats. The differences in digestive morphology and physiology underscore the evolutionary adaptations of species to their specific diets.

Digestive Physiology: The physiological processes of digestion involve multiple coordinated actions, including ingestion, mechanical breakdown, chemical digestion, absorption, and elimination. The process begins with the voluntary act of ingestion, where food is taken into the mouth. Mechanical breakdown occurs through mastication, followed by mixing with saliva, which begins enzymatic digestion. Once food is swallowed, it enters the esophagus, where peristaltic movements propel it toward the stomach. In the stomach, food is mixed with gastric juices, leading to the formation of chyme, a semi-liquid mixture that further undergoes enzymatic digestion. The chyme then enters the small intestine, where bile and pancreatic juices are secreted to facilitate fat emulsification and the digestion of carbohydrates and proteins. Absorption occurs primarily in the jejunum and ileum, where nutrients are transported into the bloodstream or lymphatic system for distribution throughout the body. The large intestine plays a crucial role in water absorption and waste compaction. The fermentation of indigestible materials by gut microbiota in species such as horses and rabbits contributes to energy recovery and nutrient synthesis, demonstrating the importance of microbial symbiosis in the digestive process.

The Role of Gut Microbiota: Recent advances in veterinary science have highlighted the importance of gut microbiota in digestive health. The microbial community residing in the gastrointestinal tract influences digestion, nutrient absorption, and immune function. Dysbiosis, or an imbalance in gut microbiota, can lead to gastrointestinal diseases and systemic health issues. In ruminants, for example, the balance of microbial populations in the rumen is crucial for effective fermentation of fibrous feeds. Disruptions in this balance can lead to metabolic disorders such as acidosis or laminitis. Understanding the interactions between diet, gut microbiota, and digestive physiology is essential for maintaining optimal health in veterinary patients.

Conclusion: The digestive system is a vital and intricate component of veterinary anatomy, essential for the survival and health of animals. Its complex structure, particularly the four compartments of the ruminant stomach, and specialized functions reflect the diverse dietary adaptations across species. A comprehensive understanding of digestive anatomy and physiology is critical for veterinary practitioners, enabling them to diagnose and treat gastrointestinal disorders effectively, manage nutritional needs, and appreciate the role of gut microbiota in overall health. As research continues to evolve in this field, it enhances our ability to ensure the well-being of animals and optimize their dietary management.

Multiple Choice Questions

1. The opening of fore-gut into mid-gut is called portal_________.
   a) Anterior intestinal b) Posterior intestinal
   c) Venous d) Foramen caecum
2. The opening of hind-gut into mid-gut is called portal__________.
   a) Anterior intestinal b) Posterior intestinal
   c) Venous d) Foramen caecum
3. Mid-gut remains continuous with the extra-embryonic_________.
   a) Allantois b) Chorion
   c) Amnion d) Yolk sac
4. oropharyngeal membrane is formed by apposition of pharyngeal endoderm and oral_____________.
   a) Ectoderm b) Gill cleft
   c) Mesoderm d) Both a & c
5. Cloacal membrane or anal plate is formed by apposition of hind-gut endoderm and
   a) Gill cleft b) Superficial ectoderm
   c) Mesoderm d) Both b & c
6. The intramural glands of the gut wall are derived from.
   a) Endoderm b) Ectoderm
   c) Mesoderm d) Both a and b

7. Both the digestive and urogenital systems open into embryonic.
   a) Rectum b) Cloaca
   c) Anus d) Proctodeum
8. Embryonic cloaca splits into rectum and
   a) Urogenital sinus b) Cloaca
   c) Anus d) None of these
9. Fore gut develops into all structures from to descending duodenum.
   a) Urogenital sinus b) Oesophagus
   c) Anus d) Pharynx
10. Mid-gut develops into all structures from to part of transverse colon.
   a) Ascending duodenum b) Descending duodenum
   c) Colon d) Jejunum
11. Hind-gut develops into all structures of transverse colon in part to
   a) Anus b) Caecum
   c) Rectum d) None of these
12. Most of the salivary glands develop from
   a) Mesoderm b) Endoderm
   c) Ectoderm d) Both a & c
13. which one is a paired lingual primordium.
   a) Lateral b) Median
   c) Proximal d) All of the above
14. the greater and lesser omentum develop from mesoderm.
   a) Somatic b) Paraxial
   c) Intermediate d) Splanchnic
15. Liver develops from.
   a) Mesoderm b) Ectoderm
   c) Endoderm d) None of these
16. Pancreas develops from.
   a) Mesoderm b) Ectoderm
   c) Endoderm d) None of these
17. Cells of the islets of Langerhans in pancreas develop from.
   a) Mesoderm b) Ectoderm
   c) Endoderm d) None of these
18. spleen is developed from.
   a) Mesoderm b) Ectoderm
   c) Endoderm d) None of these
19. omentum is developed from.
   a) Mesoderm b) Ectoderm
   c) Endoderm d) None of these

20. Cloacal membrane is formed by fusion of hind gut endoderm and
    a) Mesoderm b) Neural crest
    c) Surface ectoderm d) None of these
21. Which folds splits the embryonic cloaca into rectum and urogenital sinus
    a) Uro rectal b) Genital
    c) Cloacal d) None of these
22. Tissue develops further that lie between anal and urogenital membranes
    a) Perineum b) Penis
    c) Anus d) Urinary bladder
23. Pharyngeal pouches are in number
    a) 2 b) 6
    c) 8 d) 4 to 5
24. Left umbilical vein of the fetus runs through the .
    a) Falciform ligament b) Round ligament of liver
    c) Coronary ligament d) Lesser omentum
25. The duct from the ventral pancreatic primordium forms the.
    a) Pancreatic duct b) Common bile duct
    c) Accessory pancreatic duct d) Bile duct
26. The duct from the dorsal pancreatic primordium forms the
    a) Accessory pancreatic duct b) Pancreatic duct
    c) Common bile duct d) Bile duct
27. Both pancreatic and accessory pancreatic ducts are seen in
    a) Dog c) Cattle
    b) Cat d) Fowl
28. Accessory pancreatic ducts are seen in.
    a) Dog b) Cattle
    c) Pig d) Both b & c
29. Sheep has only one duct of pancreas called
    a) Pancreatic duct b) Common bile duct
    c) Bile duct d) Both a & b
30. Hepatic primordium develops as ventral growth from the presumptive cranial part of.
    a) Jejunum b) Duodenum
    c) Stomach d) Pancreas
31. Vascular channel between the vein and the hepatic part of posterior vena cava forms ductus venosus
    a) Left umbilical b) Right umbilical
    c) Umbilical d) Inguinal

32. Epithelium of gall bladder originates from
    a) Endoderm b) Mesoderm
    c) Ectoderm d) Neural crest
33. Body of tongue develops from.
    a) Distal lingual primordial b) Copula
    c) Median lingual primordial d) Both a & c
34. Root of tongue develops from.
    a) Distal lingual primordial b) Copula
    c) Median lingual primordial d) Both a & c
35. Dental laminae are derived from
    a) Endoderm b) Mesoderm
    c) Ectoderm d) Neural crest
36. Tooth primordium are derived from
    a) Endoderm b) Mesoderm
    c) Ectoderm d) Neural crest
37. Dental bud are derived from
    a) Endoderm b) Mesoderm
    c) Ectoderm d) Neural crest
38. The mesenchymal cells present in dental papilla originates from
    a) Endoderm b) Mesoderm
    c) both b & d d) Neural crest
40. Ameloblasts that produce enamel of tooth originates from.
    a) Endoderm b) Mesoderm
    c) Ectoderm d) Neural crest
41. Cementoblasts of tooth develops from
    a) Endoderm b) Mesoderm
    c) Ectoderm d) Neural crest
42. Odontoblasts of tooth develops from
    a) Endoderm b) Mesoderm
    c) Ectoderm d) Neural crest
43. Guttural pouch of horse develops from pharyngeal pouch.
    a) 1st b) 2nd
    c) 3rd d) 4th
44. In mammals which pharyngeal pouch is rudimentary
    a) 1st b) 2nd
    c) 3rd d) 5th
45. Paletine fossa is formed by pharyngeal pouch.
    a) 1st b) 2nd
    c) 3rd d) 5th

Answer Key

1	a	2	b	3	d	4	d	5	d	6	a	7	b
8	a	9	d	10	a	11	c	12	c	13	a	14	d
15	c	16	c	17	c	18	a	19	a	20	c	21	a
22	a	23	d	24	a	25	a	26	a	27	a	28	
29	a	30	b	31	a	32	a	33	d	34	b	35	c
36	c	37	c	38	c	39	c	40	c	41	c	42	d
43	a	44	d	45	b								

18

Development of Respiratory System

Dangeti V.V.N.D. Prasa D.[1], Ratnesh Kr. Choudhary[2], M.P.S. Tomar[3] and K. Archana[3]

[1]*Assistant Professor, Section of Veterinary Anatomy, ICAR-IVRI, Izatnagar, Bareilly Uttar Pradesh*

[2]*Associate Professor, Department of Veterinary Anatomy, BVC, BASU, Patna, Bihar*

[3]*Assistant Professor, Department of Veterinary Anatomy Sri Venkateswara Veterinary University, Tirupati, Andhra Pradesh*

Introduction

The development of the respiratory system in animals is a crucial process that begins early during embryogenesis. The respiratory system, responsible for gas exchange, develops from the endoderm of the early embryo, which is one of the three germ layers. Specifically, the respiratory tract develops as an outgrowth from the primitive gut tube (foregut). This process involves complex interactions of molecular signalling, tissue differentiation, and organ morphogenesis.

Key Stages of Respiratory System Development

1. Formation of the Respiratory Primordium

The respiratory system originates from the laryngotracheal groove, which appears on the ventral wall of the primitive foregut.

This groove eventually forms the laryngotracheal tube, which serves as the foundation for the respiratory tract.

2. Division of the Foregut

The foregut is divided into two regions:

The dorsal portion (oesophagus) for the digestive system.

The ventral portion (laryngotracheal tube) for the respiratory system.

This separation is achieved by the formation of the tracheoesophageal septum.

3. Development of the Trachea and Lung Buds

The laryngotracheal tube elongates and gives rise to the trachea)

At its distal end, two lung buds form, which will develop into the bronchi and lungs.

These lung buds expand, branch, and grow into the surrounding mesenchyme, a process called branching morphogenesis.

4. Bronchial Tree Formation

The lung buds divide into two primary bronchi, which further divide into secondary and tertiary bronchi, forming the bronchial tree.

This process is species-specific and determines the structure of the respiratory tract in various animals (e.g., lobular pattern in mammals).

5. Alveolar Development

The final stage involves the development of alveoli, the tiny air sacs where gas exchange occurs.

The alveoli form during the later stages of gestation and may continue to develop after birth in certain animals.

Species Variations

While the general process of respiratory embryology is conserved, species differences exist in timing, branching patterns, and complexity of the lungs.

Mammals have well-developed alveolar lungs.

Birds develop a highly efficient respiratory system with air sacs in addition to the lungs.

Reptiles and amphibians have simpler lung structures with less branching.

Conclusion: The embryological development of the respiratory system is a coordinated and sequential process involving endodermal and mesodermal tissues, guided by specific signalling pathways (e.g., FGF, BMP, and SHH). The resulting structures enable efficient gas exchange necessary for survival after birth or hatching, with adaptations tailored to each species' lifestyle and environment.

Multiple Choice Questions

1. The respiratory system in mammals develops from which embryonic germ layer?
   a) Ectoderm b) Endoderm
   c) Mesoderm d) All of the above
2. The lungs arise from which part of the embryonic foregut?
   a) Pharyngeal pouch b) Ventral wall
   c) Dorsal wall d) Hindgut
3. The laryngotracheal groove appears during which week of mammalian development?
   a) 2nd week b) 3rd week
   c) 4th week d) 5th week
4. The trachea and esophagus are separated by the:
   a) Tracheoesophageal ridge b) Bronchial fold
   c) Foregut partition d) Pleuroperitoneal membrane
5. Which signaling pathway is primarily involved in lung branching morphogenesis?
   a) Sonic Hedgehog (Shh) b) Wnt
   c) BMP d) All of the above
6. Lung buds begin to form during which stage of embryonic development?
   a) Pre-acinar b) Embryonic stage
   c) Pseudo glandular stage d) Canalicular stage

7. How many primary bronchial buds form initially?
   a) 1 b) 2
   c) 3 d) 4
8. The alveoli continue developing postnatally until the age of:
   a) 1 year b) 2 years
   c) 8 years d) 12 years
9. Which of the following is the last stage in lung development?
   a) Pseudo glandular stage b) Canalicular stage
   c) Alveolar stage d) Saccular stage
10. The epithelial lining of the respiratory tract is derived from:
   a) Endoderm b) Mesoderm
   c) Ectoderm d) Neural crest cells
11. The cartilages of the larynx are derived from:
   a) Endoderm
   b) Mesoderm of the pharyngeal arches
   c) Neural crest cells
   d) Surface ectoderm
12. During the pseudo glandular stage, the developing lung resembles:
   a) Mature alveoli b) Tubular glands
   c) Bronchioles with capillary networks d) Gas-exchanging sacs
13. The fetal lung produces surfactant starting around which week of development?
   a) 20th week b) 22nd week
   c) 24th week d) 28th week
14. The pleural cavities are formed by the division of which embryonic structure?
   a) Pericardial cavity b) Peritoneal cavity
   c) Intraembryonic coelom d) Neural canal
15. The diaphragm develops from all the following structures EXCEPT:
   a) Septum transversum b) Pleuroperitoneal membranes
   c) Dorsal mesentery of the esophagus d) Ectodermal placode
16. What is the role of surfactant in the fetal lungs?
   a) Prevents airway collapse b) Aids in gas exchange
   c) Lowers surface tension d) All of the above
17. The canalicular stage of lung development is characterized by:
   a) Formation of terminal sacs b) Vascularization of the lung tissue
   c) Branching of the airway tree d) Surfactant production
18. The first breath of a newborn mammal expands which structure?
   a) Alveoli b) Trachea
   c) Bronchi d) Pleural cavity

19. Which cells in the lungs produce surfactant?
    a) Type I alveolar cells
    b) Type II alveolar cells
    c) Goblet cells
    d) Club cells
20. What is the primary defect in tracheoesophageal fistula?
    a) Incomplete lung lobes
    b) Failure of the tracheoesophageal septum to form
    c) Excess surfactant production
    d) Diaphragm herniation
21. At what stage does the respiratory diverticulum (lung bud) appear?
    a) 2nd week
    b) 4th week
    c) 6th week
    d) 8th week
22. The respiratory diverticulum arises as an outgrowth of the:
    a) Hindgut
    b) Foregut
    c) Midgut
    d) Cloaca
23. The separation of the trachea and esophagus occurs during which week of development?
    a) 3rd week
    b) 4th week
    c) 5th week
    d) 6th week
24. The splanchnic mesoderm surrounding the developing lungs gives rise to:
    a) Epithelial lining of bronchi
    b) Cartilage, muscles, and connective tissues
    c) Alveolar epithelium
    d) Pleural cavity lining
25. Which molecular signaling factor is crucial for the initial formation of the respiratory system?
    a) Fibroblast Growth Factor 10 (FGF10)
    b) Sonic Hedgehog (Shh)
    c) Bone Morphogenetic Protein (BMP)
    d) Notch
26. The canalicular stage of lung development occurs during which weeks?
    a) 5th–16th weeks
    b) 16th–26th weeks
    c) 26th–36th weeks
    d) Postnatal period
27. Deficiency of surfactant in premature infants leads to which condition?
    a) Bronchitis
    b) Respiratory Distress Syndrome (RDS)
    c) Asthma
    d) Pneumonia
28. Which structure separates the pleural and pericardial cavities?
    a) Pleuropericardial folds
    b) Septum transversum
    c) Peritoneum
    d) Dorsal mesentery

29. Which transcription factor is vital for the differentiation of lung epithelial cells?
    a) TTF-1 (Thyroid Transcription Factor 1)
    b) Pax6
    c) Hox genes
    d) Oct4
30. The development of alveoli primarily occurs during the:
    a) Pseudo glandular stage b) Canalicular stage
    c) Saccular stage d) Alveolar stage
31. The larynx develops from which pharyngeal arches?
    a) First and second b) Third and fourth
    c) Fourth and sixth d) Fifth and sixth
32. What separates the nasal cavity from the oral cavity during development?
    a) Septum transversum b) Nasal septum
    c) Palatine shelves d) Pleuropericardial membrane
33. The conducting airways are fully formed during which stage of lung development?
    a) Pseudo glandular stage b) Embryonic stage
    c) Saccular stage d) Alveolar stage
34. The alveolar sacs in the fetal lung are lined by:
    a) Type I pneumocytes only
    b) Type II pneumocytes only
    c) Both Type I and Type II pneumocytes
    d) Ciliated epithelium
35. The pleura surrounding the lungs is derived from:
    a) Splanchnic mesoderm b) Somatic mesoderm
    c) Endoderm d) Ectoderm
36. Which week marks the beginning of surfactant production in human fetal lungs?
    a) 16th week b) 20th week
    c) 24th week d) 28th week
37. Which of the following disorders results from incomplete separation of the trachea and esophagus?
    a) Respiratory Distress Syndrome b) Tracheoesophageal fistula
    c) Congenital diaphragmatic hernia d) Bronchopulmonary dysplasia
38. At birth, the lungs transition from a fluid-filled organ to one used for gas exchange because of:
    a) Surfactant production b) Removal of alveolar fluid
    c) First breath inflation d) All of the above
39. The bronchioles are formed during which stage of lung development?
    a) Pseudo glandular stage b) Canalicular stage
    c) Saccular stage d) Alveolar stage

40. The diaphragm is primarily derived from which structure?
    a) Septum transversum b) Pleuroperitoneal folds
    c) Dorsal mesentery of esophagus d) All of the above
41. Which signaling pathway determines the proximal-distal patterning of the lung airways?
    a) Sonic Hedgehog (Shh) b) Fibroblast Growth Factor (FGF)
    c) Bone Morphogenetic Protein (BMP) d) Notch
42. What is the role of Sonic Hedgehog (Shh) in the branching morphogenesis of the lungs?
    a) Promotes mesodermal proliferation
    b) Inhibits epithelial branching in the distal lung bud
    c) Regulates separation of trachea and esophagus
    d) Activates Wnt signaling in airway epithelial cells
43. How does FGF10 influence lung development?
    a) Guidesbranching morphogenesis by acting as a chemoattractant for epithelial cells
    b) Regulates differentiation of alveolar cells
    c) Promotes vascular development in the lungs
    d) Inhibits mesenchymal cell proliferation
44. Which transcription factor is critical for the formation of lung epithelial progenitor cells?
    a) SOX2 b) NKX2.1
    c) TTF-1 d) PAX6
45. Which molecular interaction prevents premature branching of lung buds during development?
    a) BMP inhibition by Noggin b) FGF10 inhibition by Shh
    c) Wnt signaling inhibition by BMP d) Shh inhibition by FGF10
46. The vascularization of the developing lung begins during which stage?
    a) Embryonic stage b) Pseudoglandular stage
    c) Canalicular stage d) Saccular stage
47. The diaphragm's central tendon forms from which embryonic structure?
    a) Septum transversum b) Pleuropericardial membrane
    c) Dorsal mesentery of the esophagus d) Splanchnic mesoderm
48. Which gene is essential for the specification of the respiratory endoderm?
    a) NKX2.1 b) FOXA2
    c) SOX17 d) GATA4
49. What embryonic abnormality causes congenital diaphragmatic hernia (CDH)?
    a) Incomplete fusion of the pleuroperitoneal folds
    b) Failure of tracheoesophageal septum formation
    c) Insufficient surfactant production
    d) Disruption of Shh signaling

50. Alveolar Type I and Type II cells differentiate under the influence of which factor?
   a) TGF-β (Transforming Growth Factor Beta)
   b) BMP4 (Bone Morphogenetic Protein 4)
   c) Glucocorticoids
   d) VEGF (Vascular Endothelial Growth Factor)

51. Which germ layer gives rise to the lungs?
   a) Ectoderm
   b) Mesoderm
   c) Endoderm
   d) Both mesoderm and endoderm

52. What is the initial structure from which the lungs develop?
   a) Trachea
   b) Laryngotracheal groove
   c) Bronchial tree
   d) Pleural cavity

53. During which stage do the terminal bronchioles develop?
   a) Embryonic
   b) Pseudoglandular
   c) Canalicular
   d) Alveolar

54. What marks the transition from the canalicular to the saccular stage?
   a) Formation of the trachea
   b) Appearance of alveolar sacs
   c) Formation of primary bronchi
   d) Formation of the pleural cavity

55. The type I alveolar cells are derived from which precursor?
   a) Endodermal epithelial cells
   b) Mesenchymal cells
   c) Neural crest cells
   d) Myoblasts

56. Type II alveolar cells secrete what substance?
   a) Surfactant
   b) Mucus
   c) Hemoglobin
   d) Elastin

57. The production of surfactant increases significantly during which stage of lung development?
   a) Pseudo glandular
   b) Canalicular
   c) Saccular
   d) Alveolar

58. The alveolar stage continues postnatally in humans until what age?
   a) 1 month
   b) 6 months
   c) 2 years
   d) 8 years

59. What percentage of the alveoli are formed postnatally?
   a) 20%
   b) 40%
   c) 60%
   d) 80%

60. Which structure becomes the conducting airway in adults?
   a) Alveolar ducts
   b) Terminal bronchioles
   c) Respiratory bronchioles
   d) Trachea and bronchi

61. At which week of human gestation does the pseudoglandular stage end?
   a) 10 weeks
   b) 16 weeks
   c) 24 weeks
   d) 32 weeks

62. The term "bronchopulmonary dysplasia" refers to:
   a) A congenital anomaly in lung branching
   b) Chronic lung disease in premature infants
   c) Malformation of the bronchi
   d) Genetic mutation in lung development

63. What is Laryngococele characterized by?
   a) Abnormal lung fissures
   b) Underdeveloped lung tissue
   c) Enlarged laryngeal cavity
   d) Thoracic wall defect

64. What is Agenesis and hypoplasia of the lung?
   a) Overdevelopment of lung tissue
   b) Abnormal lung fissures
   c) Underdevelopment or absence of lung tissue
   d) Lung hernia

65. What is a possible cause of Lung hernia?
   a) Abnormal lung fissures
   b) Underdeveloped lung tissue
   c) Defect in the thoracic wall
   d) Enlarged laryngeal cavity

66. What anomaly involves the formation of unusual lung divisions?
   a) Laryngococele
   b) Lung hernia
   c) Agenesis and hypoplasia
   d) Abnormal fissures or accessory lobe

67. What is the primary cause of Hare lip?
   a) Abnormal nasal pits
   b) Non-fusion of lateral and medial nasal processes, frontonasal process, etc)
   c) Mandibular defect
   d) Congenital fistula

68. What is Congenital fistula often caused by?
   a) Non-fusion of mandibular processes
   b) Formation of abnormal nasal pits
   c) Hare lip
   d) Middle mandibular defect

69. What anomaly occurs due to non-fusion of mandibular processes?
   a) Hare lip
   b) Congenital fistula
   c) Middle mandibular defect
   d) Abnormal nasal pits

70. Which of the following is a characteristic of mandible development in cattle?
   a) Mandibles fuse completely in adult life
   b) Mandibles never fuse
   c) Mandibles form a symphysis in adult life
   d) Mandibles are absent

71. In domestic mammals, how many lobar bronchi does the right principal bronchus typically divide into?
    a) 2
    b) 3
    c) 4
    d) 5
72. In domestic mammals, how many lobar bronchi does the left principal bronchus typically divide into?
    a) 2
    b) 3
    c) 4
    d) 5
73. Which lobe is absent in horses?
    a) Cranial lobe
    b) Middle lobe
    c) Caudal lobe
    d) Accessory lobe
74. In ruminants and swine, which bronchus supplies the right cranial lobe?
    a) Principal bronchus
    b) Lobar bronchus
    c) Tracheal bronchus
    d) Bronchioles
75. What is the embryonic origin of the epithelium lining the nasal cavity?
    a) Endoderm
    b) Ectoderm
    c) Mesoderm
    d) Neural crest cells
76. Which embryonic layer gives rise to the epithelium lining the rest of the respiratory system (excluding the nasal cavity)?
    a) Ectoderm
    b) Endoderm
    c) Mesoderm
    d) Neural crest cells
77. What is the difference in embryonic origin between the epithelium lining the nasal cavity and the rest of the respiratory system?
    a) Both are derived from ectoderm
    b) Both are derived from endoderm
    c) Nasal cavity epithelium is from ectoderm, while the rest of the respiratory system is from endoderm
    d) Nasal cavity epithelium is from endoderm, while the rest of the respiratory system is from ectoderm
78. How are the paranasal sinuses initially formed?
    a) From mesenchymal growths into the nasal cavity
    b) From epithelial growths into the mesenchyme of the nasal cavity walls
    c) From the conchae directly
    d) From the maxillae bones
79. What structure do the maxillary sinuses develop from?
    a) Frontal sinuses
    b) Ethmoidal conchae
    c) Diverticula expanding into the maxillae walls
    d) Nasal cavity directly

80. How do the frontal sinuses typically develop?
   a) From the rostral part of the nasal cavity
   b) From diverticula branching from the caudal part of the nasal cavity
   c) Directly from the ethmoidal conchae
   d) From the maxillary sinuses

81. What is characteristic of paranasal sinus development at birth?
   a) They are fully formed
   b) They are partially formed
   c) They are poorly formed
   d) They are absent

82. In pigs and ruminants, what happens to the frontal sinuses throughout life?
   a) They remain constant in size
   b) They decrease in size
   c) They enlarge and influence skull morphogenesis
   d) They disappear

83. What forms the conchae in the nasal cavity?
   a) Transverse ridges on the nasal cavity wall
   b) Longitudinal ridges or laminae on the nasal cavity wall
   c) Cartilage from the nasal septum
   d) Mesenchyme from the maxillary process

84. What are the bony portions of the conchae called?
   a) Turbinates
   b) Meatuses
   c) Sinuses
   d) Nasal septum

85. What is the origin of the caudal parts of the dorsal nasal conchae?
   a) Maxillary process
   b) Ethmoid cartilages (dorsolateral parts)
   c) Mesenchyme of the nasal cavity walls
   d) Nasal septum

86. What is the developmental origin of the ventral nasal conchae?
   a) Ethmoid cartilages
   b) Maxillary process
   c) Dorsal nasal conchae
   d) Nasal septum

87. What is continuous with the ethmoidal cartilage?
   a) Mesenchyme of the nasal cavity walls
   b) Cartilage forming nasal septum and turbinates
   c) Maxillary process
   d) Nasal conchae

88. How do the longitudinal ridges or laminae affect the nasal cavity?
   a) They merge to form a single passageway
   b) They compartmentalize it into several passageways (meatuses)
   c) They form the nasal septum
   d) They create the sinuses

89. What is the developmental relationship between the rostral parts of the dorsal nasal conchae and the maxillary process?
   a) They are unrelated
   b) They are developmentally related
   c) They replace each other
   d) They fuse together

90. What determines the external shape of nasal cartilages?
   a) Species characteristics
   b) Individual characteristics
   c) Age
   d) Sex

91. What forms the vomeronasal organ?
   a) Outgrowths of nasal epithelium
   b) Ingrowths of nasal epithelium
   c) Differentiation of nasal septum
   d) Development of olfactory nerve

92. Where do the bilateral ingrowths of nasal epithelium occur?
   a) Caudal part of the nasal cavity
   b) Nasal turbinates
   c) Rostral part of the nasal septum
   d) Maxillary sinuses

93. What type of epithelium differentiates in the vomeronasal organ?
   a) Respiratory epithelium
   b) Sensory epithelium
   c) Squamous epithelium
   d) Columnar epithelium

94. What is characteristic of the sensory epithelium in the vomeronasal organ?
   a) Only supporting cells
   b) Only neurons
   c) Supporting cells and neurons
   d) No olfactory nerve

95. When is differentiation of nasal epithelium apparent?
   a) Late fetal stage
   b) Early fetal stage
   c) Postnatal development
   d) Adult life

96. What is consistent across domestic mammals regarding palate formation?
   a) Extent of palatine process fusion
   b) Basic pattern of palate formation
   c) Nasal septum development
   d) Choanae formation

97. In pigs and horses, how far caudally do palatine processes fuse with the nasal septum?
   a) Up to the choanae
   b) Beyond the internal nares
   c) To the caudal extent of the internal nares
   d) Not at all

98. What is unique about the pig's palatine shelf fusion?
   a) It extends into the nasopharynx
   b) It stops at the choanae
   c) It doesn't fuse with the nasal septum
   d) It forms a single common opening

99. In dogs and cats, where does palatine process fusion with the nasal septum typically end?
   a) Caudal extent of internal nares
   b) Rostralmost part of nasopharynx
   c) Just rostral to the choanae
   d) Not at all

100. What is characteristic of ruminants' palatine process fusion?
   a) Extensive fusion with nasal septum
   b) Fusion only up to choanae
   c) Least extent of fusion with nasal septum
   d) No fusion

Answer Key

1	b	2	b	3	c	4	a	5	d	6	b	7	b
8	c	9	c	10	a	11	b	12	b	13	c	14	c
15	d	16	d	17	b	18	a	19	b	20	b	21	b
22	b	23	b	24	b	25	a	26	b	27	b	28	a
29	a	30	d	31	c	32	b	33	a	34	c	35	a
36	c	37	b	38	d	39	a	40	d	41	b	42	c
43	a	44	b	45	b	46	c	47	a	48	a	49	a
50	c	51	d	52	b	53	b	54	b	55	a	56	a
57	d	58	d	59	d	60	d	61	b	62	b	63	c
64	c	65	c	66	d	67	b	68	b	69	c	70	c
71	c	72	a	73	b	74	c	75	b	76	b	77	c
78	b	79	c	80	b	81	c	82	c	83	b	84	a
85	b	86	b	87	b	88	b	89	b	90	a	91	b
92	c	93	b	94	c	95	b	96	b	97	c	98	a
99	c	100	c										

19

Embryology: Urinary System

K. Archana[1], Ratnesh Kr. Choudhary[2], M.P.S. Tomar[1] and Dangeti V.V.N. Durga Prasad[3]

[1]*Assistant Professor, Department of Veterinary AnatomyAnatomy Sri Venkateswara Veterinary University, Tirupati*

[2]*Associate Professor, Department of Veterinary Anatomy, BVC, BASU, Patna*

[3]*Assistant Professor, Section of Veterinary Anatomy, ICAR-IVRI, Izatnagar, Bareilly*

Introduction

The urinary system comprises of two kidneys, two ureters, a urinary bladder, and a urethra) The latter is shared by the genital organs.

- The urinary system develops from the intermediate mesoderm
- Three different kidney systems are formed in vertebrates--pronephros, mesonephros, and metanephros.

Pronephros: - Forms a duct that empties into the cloaca- Pronephric tubules connect each body segment with the coelom (body cavity)

Pronephric tubules never become functional in mammals

Mesonephros: - Pronephric duct becomes mesonephric duct

Distal to the pronephric tubules appear mesonephric tubules that surround tufts of blood vessels (glomeruli), but no loop of Henle is formed

Blood is transported to mesonephric tubules, filtrate is transported to the mesonephric duct and finally to the urogenital portion of the cloaca

Metanephros: - Metanephric bud (ureteric bud)

Metanephric blastema

- Bud gives rise to the ureter, the pelvis of the kidney, and collecting tubules.
- Blastema gives rise to nephrons.

The internal structure of the kidney varies among species. It is determined by the number and size of calyces which branch from the renal pelvis. Each calyx forms the base of a renal lobe (renal pyramid). All mammalian kidneys begin as multipyramidal (multilobular) structures, but lobules fuse to varying degrees, depending upon the species. (Note, this multilobulation is maintained in the histological structures)

Development of the Bladder and Urethra

The cloaca is subdivided caudally by the mesenchymal tissue called the urorectal septum - the dorsal part becomes the rectum and the ventral part becomes the urogenital sinus.

The urogenital sinus (U.G.S) is demarcated into the vesicular part, the urethral part, the pelvic part, and the phallic part. The urethrovesicular part expands rapidly and incorporates the distal part of the mesonephric ducts and the proximal parts of the metanephric buds (ureters). The result is that the mesonephric ducts and the ureters have separate openings into the U.G. S. The ureter enters the vesicular part which, in turn, develops into the urinary bladder.

The urethral, pelvic and phallic parts of the U.G.S. form parts of the genital systems which are discussed later.

Anomalies of the Urinary System

Hydronephrosis: Replacement of one or both kidneys with fluid-filled cysts. This is more common in dogs and sheep. It is caused by a blockage in the collecting system; mainly results from the malformation of the ureter.

Urachal Fistula (Patent Urachus): This results from the failure of the allantoic stalk to close at birth. Result: constant dribbling from the urachus.

Ectopic Ureter: This results from the malpositioning of the ureter which opens into the urethra instead of the bladder. Result: constant dribbling in females, but the incontinence does not occur in males because the ureter opens into the urethra proximal to the urethralis muscle which can voluntarily/involuntarily constrict the urethral opening.

Multiple Choice Questions

1. The urinary system of the vertebrates mostly develops from
   a) Ectoderm b) Intermediate mesoderm
   c) Lateral plate mesoderm d) Somites
2. The enzyme produced by kidney which helps in regulation of blood pressure is
   a) Renin b) Lipase
   c) Trypsin d) Amylase
3. Angiotensinogenase is the other name for
   a) Trypsin b) Lipase
   c) Renin d) Amylase
4. The cells in the kidney responsible for production of renin are
   a) Podocytes b) Juxtaglomerular cells
   c) PCT d) None
5. Erythropoeitin is produced by
   a) Hilar region b) Renal cortex
   c) Renal medulla d) Not specific
6. The pronephric tubules are located in the
   a) Cervical region b) Thoracic region
   c) Lumbar region d) Not specific

7. The mesonephric tubules are located in the
   a) Cervical region b) Sacral region
   c) Thoraco lumbar region d) Not specific
8. The metanephric tubules are located in the
   a) Cervical region b) Thoraco lumbar region
   c) Sacral region d) Not specific
9. The definitive functional kidney in fishes and amphibians
   a) Pronephros b) Mesonephros
   c) Metanephros d) None of the above
10. The definitive functional kidney in reptiles
   a) Pronephros b) Mesonephros
   c) Metanephros d) None of the above
11. The definitive functional kidney in aves
   a) Pronephros b) Mesonephros
   c) Metanephros d) None of the above
12. The definitive functional kidney in mammals
   a) Pronephros b) Mesonephros
   c) Metanephros d) None of the above
13. Pronephric tubules are first formed in the somites of this region
   a) Cervical region b) Thoracic region
   c) Lumbar region d) Coccygeal region
14. The pronephric duct opens into
   a) Rectum b) Crop
   c) Cloaca d) Caecum
15. Nephrocoele communicates with coelomic cavity through
   a) cloaca b) Nephrotome
   c) Nephrostome d) No communication
16. Cords of cells growing from the dorsal wall of the intermediate mesoderm and form pronephric tubules are called
   a) Cloaca b) Nephrotomes
   c) Nephrostome d) No communication
17. The primitive glomeruli are tufts of capillaries arising from
   a) Dorsal aorta b) Umbillical artery
   c) CBCT d) Coronary arteries
18. Glomeruli which invaginate into coelomic epithelium are referred to as
   a) Internal glomeruli b) External glomeruli
   c) Dorsal glomeruli d) None
19. Glomeruli which invaginate into coelomic epithelium are referred to as
   a) Internal glomeruli b) External glomeruli
   c) Dorsal glomeruli d) None

20. The invaginated epithelium surrounding each glomerulus is termed as
    a) Podocytes b) Bowmans capsule
    c) Distal convoluted tubule d) Proximal convoluted tubule
21. The presence of internal glomeruli is a feature of
    a) Higher vertebrates b) Lower vertebrates
    c) Both d) None
22. The presence of external glomeruli is a feature of
    a) Higher vertebrates b) Lower vertebrates
    c) Both d) None
23. The urogenital ridge develops in the thoracolumbar region of the foetus by the proliferation of
    a) Ectoderm b) Lateral plate mesoderm
    c) Intermediate mesoderm d) Endoderm
24. The urogenital ridge divides into
    a) Medial genital ridge and lateral urinary ridge
    b) Does not divide
    c) Medial genital ridge and lateral pulmonary ridge
    d) Lateral genital ridge and medial urinary ridge
25. S - shaped tubules are formed in
    a) Urinary ridge b) Genital ridge
    c) Ectoderm d) Endoderm
26. Invagination of the glomerular tuft into the mesonephric tubule epithelium induces the formation of
    a) Podocytes b) PCT
    c) Bowman's capsule d) DCT
27. Renal corpuscle consists of
    a) Bowman's capsule
    b) Glomerular tuft
    c) Both
    d) Mesonephric and pronephric duct
28. Development of the mesonephric system in the foetus causes atrophy of
    a) Pronephric tubules
    b) Cranial portion of the pronephric duct
    c) Both
    d) None
29. The number of pronephric tubules that develop at the level of each somite
    a) Two b) One
    c) Many d) Half

30. The number of mesonephric tubules that develop at the level of each somite
    a) Multiple b) One
    c) Two d) Half
31. The mesonephros are very prominent structures upto 35 days in the foetuses of
    a) Rodents b) Horse
    c) Pig d) Humans
32. The mesonephros in horses regresses around
    a) 58 days of gestation b) 65 days of gestation
    c) 50 days of gestation d) 36 days of gestation
33. The mesonephros in cattle regresses around
    a) 58 days of gestation b) 65 days of gestation
    c) 50 days of gestation d) 36 days of gestation
34. The mesonephros in Pigs regresses around
    a) 58 days of gestation b) 65 days of gestation
    c) 50 days of gestation d) 36 days of gestation
35. The mesonephros in Dogs regresses around
    a) 58 days of gestation b) 65 days of gestation
    c) 50 days of gestationd. d) 36 days of gestation
36. The presence of giant glomeruli associated with mesonephric tubules is a feature of
    a) Ruminant embryos b) Equine embryos
    c) Porcine embryos d) Canine embryos
37. The ureteric bud is an outgrowth of
    a) Pronephric duct b) Mesonephric duct
    c) Metanephric blastema d) B and C
38. Metanephric blastema in the embryo is located in
    a) Lumbar region b) Sacral region
    c) Thoracic region d) Coccygeal region
39. Metanephric blastema in the embryo is formed in
    a) Lateral edge of urinary ridge b) Cranial end of the nephric ridge
    c) Caudal end of the nephric ridge d) Genital ridge
40. The ureteric bud extends towards
    a) Metanephric blastema b) Cloaca
    c) Lateral wall d) ventral abdominal wall
41. Ureteric bud gives rise to
    a) Pelvis b) Collecting ducts
    c) PCT d) A and B
42. The metanephric tubules arise from
    a) Metanephric blastema b) Ureteric bud
    c) Both d) None

43. Primary inducer of ureteric bud branching is
a) Gdnf
b) Tgf-beta
c) Hgf
d) None

44. Tubular growth and branching is regulated by
a) Inhibitory growth factors
b) Tgf-beta
c) Bone morphogenic proteins
d) All

45. Factors secreted by ureteric bud cells which induce mesenchymal differentiation into leading to formation of metanephric tubules
a) FGf-2
b) Bmp-4
c) Both A and B
d) Wt-1

46. Factors responsible for differentiation of mesenchyme to epithelium are
a) Pax-2
b) Wnt-4
c) Fgf-2
d) Both A and B

47. Charecteristic component of epithelial basal laminae are
a) Laminin
b) Type IV collagen
c) Type I collagen
d) Both A and B

48. The cell adhesion molecules responsible for differentiation of mesenchyme to epithelium
a) Syndecan
b) E-cadherin
c) Both A and B
d) Temporal bone

49. The term nephron refers to
a) Renal corpuscle
b) Loop of Henle
c) Proximal and Distal convoluted tubule
d) All the above

50. The renal cortex mainly consists of
a) Renal corpuscles
b) Proximal convoluted tubule
c) Distal convoluted tubule
d) All the above

51. Medullary pyramid consists of
a) Loops of Henle
b) Collecting ducts
c) Both A and B
d) Renal corpuscles

52. The base of the renal medullary pyramid is capped by
a) Renal cortex
b Renal Medulla
c) Pelvis
d) Cloaca

53. The apex of the medullary pyramid projects into
a) Renal cortex
b) Renal Medulla
c) Pelvis
d) Cloaca

54. Unilobar kidneys are present in
a) Rodents
b) Rabbits
c) Cattle
d) Both A and B

55. Blood supply is directly from dorsal aorta in
    a) Pronephros b) Mesonephros
    c) Metanephros d) Both A and B
56. Blood supply to each nephron is from a branch of renal artery in
    a) Pronephros b) Mesonephros
    c) Metanephros d) Both A and B
57. During differentiation the position of the metanephros changes from
    a) Pelvic to lumbar region b) Pelvic to sacral region
    c) Pelvic to thoracic region d) Lumbar to pelvic region
58. In domestic animals the kidney that migrates more cranially is
    a) Left kidney b) Right kidney
    c) Both migrate at the same level d) None
59. The kidney in contact with the caudate lobe of liver is
    a) Left kidney b) Right kidney
    c) Both migrate at the same level d) None
60. Renculus is the term given to the kidney lobes of
    a) Domestic animals b) Pig
    c) Aquatic mammals d) Camel
61. The number of major branches developing from the ureter of domestic animals
    a) Two b) Multiple
    c) Three d) Four
62. Renal pelvis is absent in
    a) Bovine kidney b) Equine kidney
    c) Canine kidney d) All the above
63. Renal pelvis is present in
    a) Bovine kidney b) Equine kidney
    c) Canine kidney d) Both B and C
64. Renal crest is a charecteristic feature of
    a) Bovine kidney b) Equine kidney
    c) Canine kidney d) Both B and C
65. The kidneys give appearance of bunch of grapes in
    a) Aquatic mammals b) Bovine kidney
    c) Canine kidney d) Both B and C
66. Developmental failure of one or both ureteric buds results in
    a) Renal agenesis b) Ectopic kidney
    c) Horse shoe kidney d) Congenital cystic kidney
67. If a kidney remains in the sacral region it is referred to as
    a) Renal agenesis b) Ectopic kidney
    c) Horse shoe kidney d) Congenital cystic kidney

68. The best example proving that ontogeny repeats phylogeny is the development of
    a) Urinary system b) Respiratory system
    c) Respiratory system d) Male reproductive system
69. The order in which kidneys form during development of an individual is
    a) Mesonephros - Pronephros -metanephros
    b) Pronephros- metanephros - mesonephros
    c) Pronephros-mesonephros-metanephros
    d) Metanephros-Pronephros-mesonephros
70. The genital system develops in close association with
    a) Urinary system b) Respiratory system
    c) Respiratory system d) Male reproductive system
71. The mesonephric duct opens into
    a) Rectum b) Crop
    c) Cloaca d) caecum
72. The mesonephric system completely regresses in
    a) Males b) Females
    c) Both d) Does not develop in both
73. The mesonephric system ducts persist to form parts of the genital system in
    a) Males b) Females
    c) Both d) Does not develop in both
74. Defective partitioning of cloaca results in
    a) Rectovaginal fistula b) Urachal cyst
    c) Urachal fistula d) All the above
75. Persistence of allantois results in
    a) Urachal sinus b) Urachal cyst
    c) Urachal fistula d) All the above
76. Defective partitioning of cloaca results in
    a) Rectovaginal fistula b) Rectourethral fistula
    c) Urachal fistula d) Both A and B
77. Defective partitioning of cloaca in males results in
    a) Rectovaginal fistula b) Rectourethral fistula
    c) Urachal fistula d) Both A and B
78. Defective partitioning of cloaca in females results in
    a) Rectovaginal fistula b) Rectourethral fistula
    c) Urachal fistula d) Both A and B
79. Anomaly resulting due to fusion of cranial poles of kidney
    a) Horseshoe kidney b) Pelvic rosette kidney
    c) Urachal fistula d) Urachal cyst

80. Anomaly resulting due to fusion of caudal poles of kidney
    a) Horseshoe kidney b) Pelvic rosette kidney
    c) Urachal fistula d) Urachal cyst
81. Replacement of one or both kidneys with fluid-filled cysts
    a) Horseshoe kidney b) Pelvic rosette kidney
    c) Hydronephrosis d) Urachal cyst
82. The urorectal septum divides the cloaca into
    a) Dorsal rectum and ventral urogenital sinus.
    b) Dorsal urogenital sinus and ventral rectum.
    c) It does not divide cloaca)
    d) Dorsal urinary and ventrally rectum.
83. Failure of allantois to close resulting in dribbling of urine in newborn is due to
    a) Horseshoe kidney b) Pelvic rosette kidney
    c) Urachal fistula d) Urachal cyst
84. Functional Pronephros seen in which species
    a) Sheep b) Goat
    c) Ox d) Dog
85. Ureteric bud modifies in adult to
    a) Ureter b) Urethra
    c) Penis d) Gonads
86. Single pronephric glomeruli seen in
    a) Sheep b) Goat
    c) Ox d) Dog
87. Mesonephric glomeruli seen in
    a) Sheep b) Goat
    c) Ox d) Dog
88. Collecting ducts of kidney are derived from
    a) Metanephric mesenchyme b) Ureteric bud
    c) Wolffian duct d) Pronephros
89. Horse shoe kidney
    a) Abnormal rotation b) Fusion of Metanephric kidney
    c) Failure of Ureteric bud formation d) Failure of ascent
90. Trigone of bladder derived from
    a) Ureteric bud b) Mesonephric duct
    c) Metanephros d) Endoderm
91. Process by which the ureteric bud induces the Metanephric mesenchyme to differentiate into nephrons is called
    a) Reciprocal induction b) Apoptosis
    c) Segmentation d) Neurulation

92. The fate of tubules of mesonephros in male
    a) Metanephric kidney
    b) Efferent Ductules
    c) Testes
    d) Kidneys
93. The ascent of kidneys is initially vascularised by branches of the
    a) Aorta
    b) External Iliac
    c) Internal Iliac aretry
    d) Carotid artery
94. Renal pelvis developed from
    a) Ureteric bud
    b) Metanephric blastema
    c) Mesonephric duct
    d) Cloaca
95. Calyces are developed from
    a) Ureteric bud
    b) Metanephric blastema
    c) Mesonephric duct
    d) Cloaca
96. Collecting tubes and papillary ducts are developed from
    a) Ureteric bud
    b) Metanephric blastema
    c) Mesonephric duct
    d) Cloaca
97. Bowman's capsule derived from
    a) Ureteric bud
    b) Metanephric blastema
    c) Mesonephric duct
    d) Cloaca
98. Pol ycystic kidney Disease is primarily due to mutations
    a) Nephrogenesis
    b) Tubular Development
    c) Glomerular Formation
    d) Ureteric bud elongation
99. Duplication of ureter results from
    a) Early division of ureteric bud
    b) Failure of ureteric bud to induce mesenchyme
    c) Malrotation of kidney
    d) Incomplete ascent of kidney
100. The Pronephros disappears at the end of
    a) 2nd week
    b) 3rd week
    c) 4th week
    d) 5th week
101. The urinary bladder derived from of
    a) Cloaca
    b) Mesonephric duct
    c) Metanephric kidney
    d) Prostate
102. Allantois regress to form
    a) Urachus
    b) Ureter
    c) Trigone
    d) Renal Pelvis
103. The Patent Urachus results in
    a) Absence of one kidney
    b) Formation of cysts
    c) Blockage of urethra
    d) Leakage of urine from umbilicus

Answer Key

1	b	2	a	3	c	4	b	5	b	6	a	7	c
8	c	9	b	10	c	11	c	12	c	13	a	14	c
15	c	16	b	17	a	18	b	19	a	20	a	21	b
22	b	23	c	24	a	25	a	26	c	27	c	28	c
29	b	30	a	31	c	32	b	33	a	34	c	35	d
36	a	37	d	38	b	39	c	40	a	41	d	42	a
43	a	44	d	45	c	46	d	47	d	48	c	49	d
50	d	51	c	52	a	53	c	54	d	55	d	56	a
57	a	58	b	59	b	60	c	61	a	62	a	63	d
64	d	65	a	66	a	67	b	68	a	69	c	70	a
71	c	72	b	73	a	74	a	75	d	76	d	77	b
78	a	79	b	80	a	81	c	82	a	83	c	84	a
85	a	86	a	87	a	88	b	89	d	90	b	91	a
92	b	93	a	94	a	95	a	96	a	97	b	98	b
99	a	100	c	101	a	102	a	103	d				

20

Development of Reproductive System

Shalini Suri[1], Jasvinder Singh Sasan[1] and Yousuf Dar[2]

[1]Division of Veterinary Anatomy, Faculty of Veterinary Sciences and Animal Husbandry Sher-e-Kashmir University of Agricultural Sciences and Technology of Jammu, Jammu and Kashmir

[2]Division of Veterinary Anatomy and Histology, Faculty of Veterinary Sciences and Animal Husbandry, Sher-e-Kashmir University of Agricultural Sciences and Technology of Kashmir, Jammu and Kashmir

The presence of a Y or X chromosome influences sexual differentiation and the development of reproductive organs. The reproductive system comprises the gonads, genital ducts, external genitalia, and gonad descent. Development of reproductive system is initiated in gonads which differentiate into ovary or testis. The formation of genital ducts and glands occur later. Differentiation of reproductive system is a complex process which involves a number of different mechanisms operating at several stages of development. It occurs only after the arrival of primordial germ cells.

First, the gonads undergo an indifferent stage before differentiating into the testes and ovaries. Thereafter, the sexual differentiation of the genital ducts is determined by the presence or absence of testosterone and Anti-Müllerian hormone, both of which influence the outcome of the mesonephric and paramesonephric ducts. Then sexual distinction of the external genitalia is also determined by hormonal secretions, or lack thereof and finally, the gonads descend primarily due to the shortening of the gubernaculum.

Importantly, the development of the reproductive system is directly related to that of the urinary system. Both systems develop from common intermediate mesoderm and their excretory ducts terminate in a common cavity known as cloaca)

Two important ducts develop, i.e. wolffian duct (in males) and mullerian duct (in females). Mesonephric duct which is also known as Wolffian duct, originates from pronephric duct. Pronephric duct continues to grow caudally till it opens into the ventral part of the cloaca. Beyond pronephros (primitive kidney), it is called mesonephric duct. In males, this duct persists and forms epididymis, vas deferens and seminal vesicle. In females, this duct undergoes atrophy.

Shortly after the formation of Wolffian duct, a 2nd pair of duct develops i.e. Mullerian duct. Each arises on the lateral aspect of the corresponding Wolffian duct as a tubular invagination of the cells lining the abdominal cavity. Mullerian duct opens on cloaca between the orifices of Wolffian ducts. In females, mullerian duct persist and undergo further development.

Gonads develops from 3 important sources, namely mesothelium lining posterior abdominal wall, underlying mesenchyme (Embryonic CT) and primordial Germ Cells

External genitalia develop from 3 different perineal swellings. These are:

a) Bilateral *urogenital fold* surrounding *urogenital orifices.* Urogenital folds are caudal end of urogenital sinus

b) *Genital tubercle,* develops at ventral commissure of urogenital folds

c) Bilateral *genital/Labio-scrotal swellings.* These are located lateral to urogenital folds. In primates, these swelling develop in both sexes forming Labia major in females and scrotum in males. In domestic animals, these swellings persist in males only.

Multiple Choice Questions

1. In Females, the primordial germ cells differentiate into-
   a) Spermatogonia b) Oogonia
   c) Sertoli cells d) Leydig cells

2. The duct system of female reproductive system develops from
   a) Mullerian duct b) Mesonephric duct
   c) Wolffian duct d) None of the above

3. The mullerian duct is also known as
   a) Mesonephric duct b) Paramesonephric duct
   c) Wolffian duct d) None of the above

4. ----------------- portions of mullerian ducts become convoluted and form oviducts
   a) Cranial b) Middle
   c) Caudal d) None of the above

5. The remnants of the paramesonephric duct in males is known as
   a) Uterus musculinus (prostatic utricle) b) Gartners duct
   c) Appendix epididymis d) None of the above

6. The vestibule and vulva are developed from
   a) Mesonephric duct b) Mesonephric tubule
   c) Urogenital sinus d) None of the above

7. The remnants of the mesonephric duct in females is known as
   a) Fornix b) Gartners duct
   c) Sub urethral diverticulum d) None of the above

8. The clitoris is developed from
   a) Urogenital sinus b) Urogenital fold
   c) Genital tubercle d) None of the above

9. In ovary, the medulla is composed of degenerating intragonadal tubules known as –
   a) Corpus luteum b) Rete ovarii
   c) Granulosa cells d) None of the above

10. In mammals a high percentage of oogonia and primary oocyte undergo degenerative changes in pre and post-natal life known as –
    a) Folliculogenesis b) Oogenesis
    c) Atresia d) None of the above

11. The caudal fused portions of paramesonephric ducts form
    a) Uterus b) Cervix
    c) Cranial part of vagina d) All of the above
12. The caudal part of vagina is developed from
    a) Urogenital sinus b) Mesonephric tubule
    c) Genital tubercle d) None of the above
13. The vestibular glands are homologues to
    a) Prostate b) Vesicular glands
    c) Bulbourethral glands d) None of the above
14. The urethral glands are homologues to
    a) Prostate b) Vesicular glands
    c) Bulbourethral glands d) None of the above
15. The shape of uterus and its relationship with vagina is determined by
    a) Degeneration of mesonephric duct b) Fusion of paramesonephric duct
    c) Both d) None of the above
16. The cranial remnants of mesonephric tubules in mesovarium form
    a) Epoophoron b) Paraoophoron
    c) Rete ovarii d) None of the above
17. The caudal remnants of mesonephric tubules in mesovarium form
    a) Epoophoron b) Paraoophoron
    c) Rete ovarii d) None of the above
18. The follicles which develop from the gonadal cords are-
    a) Primordial follicles b) Primary follicles
    c) Secondary follicles t d) Tertiary follicles
19. The degree of fusion of paramesonephric ducts is high in
    a) Bovines b) Rodents
    c) Equines d) Carnivores
20. The degree of fusion of paramesonephric ducts is least in
    a) Bovines b) Rodents
    c) Equines d) Carnivores
21. In females, the genital fold forms-
    a) Mesovarium b) Mesosalphinx
    c) Mesometrium d) All of the above
22. In males, the genital fold forms-
    a) Mesorchium b) Mesoductus deferens
    c) Both d) None of the above
23. The follicles are randomly distributed in the cortex of ovary in
    a) Cattle b) Sheep
    c) Pig d) All of the above

24. The follicles are present in clusters in the cortex of ovary in
    a) Cattle b) Sheep
    c) Dog d) All of the above
25. The oogonial mitosis begins in cattle at
    a) 20 days of gestation b) 70 days of gestation
    c) 30 days of gestation d) 50 days of gestation
26. The oogonial mitosis completes in cattle at
    a) 70 days of gestation b) 90 days of gestation
    c) 110 days of gestation d) 180 days of gestation
27. Before birth, the primary oocyte begins the first meiotic division which is arrested at-
    a) Leptotene b) Zygotene
    c) Pachytene d) Diplotene
28. Before ovulation, first meiotic division is completed in
    a) Cow b) Mare
    c) Bitch d) All of the above
29. The first meiotic division is completed immediately after ovulation in
    a) Mare b) Bitch
    c) Both d) None of the above
30. The cranial vestiges of paramesonephric ducts form
    a) Prostatic utricle b) Appendix testis
    c) Gartner's duct d) All of the above
31. The primordial germ cells of gonads arise from endodermal cells of –
    a) Chorion b) Yolk sac
    c) Amnion d) Allantois
32. In males, the primordial germ cells differentiate into-
    a) Spermatogonia b) Oogonia
    c) Sertoli cells d) Leydig cells
33. In cattle, the primordial germ cells appear in genital ridges by
    a) 21 days b) 18 days
    c) 10 days d) 25 days
34. In dogs, the primordial germ cells appear in genital ridges by
    a) 21 days b) 18 days
    c) 10 days d) 28 days
35. In pigs, the primordial germ cells appear in genital ridges by
    a) 21 days b) 18 days
    c) 10 days d) 28 days
36. In Humans, the primordial germ cells appear in genital ridges by
    a) 21 days b) 18 days
    c) 10 days d) 28 days

37. In mammals, the primordial germ cells reach the genital ridge by
   a) Blood b) Active migration
   c) Both d) None of the above
38. In Avians, the primordial germ cells reach the genital ridge by
   a) Blood b) Active migration
   c) Both d) None of the above
39. The duct system of male reproductive system develops from
   a) Mesonephric tubule b) Mesonephric duct
   c) Urogenital sinus d) All of the above
40. The mesonephric duct is also known as
   a) Wolffian duct b) Mullerian duct
   c) Paramesonephric duct d) None of the above
41. The remnants of the mesonephric duct in females is known as
   a) Fornix b) Gartners duct
   c) Sub urethral diverticulum d) None of the above
42. In developing gonads, the seminiferous cords appear as
   a) Foot shaped b) Horse shoe shaped
   c) Saddle shaped d) None of the above
43. The testis are determined under the influence of
   a) Sry gene b) Srk gene
   c) X chromosome d) None of the above
44. The Sry gene is located on
   a) X chromosome b) Y chromosome
   c) Both d) None of the above
45. The Appendix testis (hydatid of Morgagni) is vestigial remnant of
   a) Mullerian duct b) Wolffian duct
   c) Both d) Urogenital sinus
46. The uterus musculinus in males is a vestigial remnant of
   a) Mullerian duct b) Wolffian duct
   c) both d) Urogenital sinus
47. Appendix epididymis is a remnant of
   a) Paramesonephric duct b) Mesonephric duct
   c) Both d) None of the above
48. The vestige of mesonephric duct cranial to developing testis is –
   a) Appendix testis b) Uterus musculinus
   c) Appendix epididymis d) None of the above
49. Some mesonephric tubules at the caudal pole of developing testis do not join with rete testis and become vestigial are known as –
   a) Epididymis b) Paradidymis
   c) Appendix testis d) Appendix epididymis

50. The prostate gland develops from
   a) Ectoderm b) Mesoderm
   c) Endoderm d) All of the above
51. The seminal vesicles develop from
   a) Ectoderm b) Endoderm
   c) Mesoderm d) None of the above
52. Bulbourethral gland develops from-
   a) Ectoderm b) Mesoderm
   c) Endoderm d) None of the above
53. The gubernaculum testis comprised of
   a) Proper ligament of testis b) Ligament of tail of epididymis
   c) Both d) None of the above
54. A fibromuscular band which extends from caudal pole of testis to the scrotum is-
   a) Epididymis b) Gubernaculum testis
   c) Rete testis d) None of the above
55. The seminiferous tubules are developed from
   a) Genital ridge b) Mesonephric tubules
   c) Mesonephric ducts d) None of the above
56. Duct of epididymis and vas deferens are developed from
   a) Genital ridge b) Mesonephric duct
   c) Urogenital sinus d) None of the above
57. The urethra (pelvic and penile) is developed from
   a) Mesonephric duct b) Mesonephric tubule
   c) Urogenital sinus d) None of the above
58. In most domestic animals testicular descent occurs before birth except
   a) Horse b) Dog
   c) Pig d) All of the above
59. In males, the inhibitory factors that suppress the paramesonephric duct are secreted by
   a) Sertoli cells b) Leydig cells
   c) Spermatogonia d) None of the above
60. In cattle, spermatogenesis occurs at
   a) 6-8 months b) 10 months
   c) 12 months d) 2 years
61. In dogs, spermatogenesis occurs at
   a) 6-8 months b) 9-10 months
   c) 12 months d) 2 years
62. In horses, spermatogenesis occurs at
   a) 6-8 months b) 9-10 months
   c) 12 months d) 2 years

63. Structure responsible for descent of testis is:
    a) Yolk sac
    b) Gubernaculum
    c) Wolffian duct
    d) Mullerian duct
64. The embryonic origin(s) of the scrotum is/are:
    a) Genital tubercle
    b) Genital swelling
    c) Urethral fold
    d) Sino-vaginal bulb
65. Genital system develops from:
    a) Par-axial mesoderm
    b) Intermediate mesoderm
    c) Notochord
    d) Lateral mesoderm
66. Which accessory sex gland/s in male develops by outgrowths of uro-genital sinus endoderm:
    a) Prostate and seminal vesicle
    b) Prostate and bulbo-urethral
    c) Seminal vesicle and bulbo-urethral
    d) Prostate, bulbo-urethral and seminal vesicle
67. Growth at the base of which of the following generates an elongate *phallus:*
    a) Uro-genital fold
    b) Genital tubercle
    c) Genital swelling
    d) Uro-genital orifice
68. Which of the following is located lateral to urogenital folds:
    a) Uro-genital fold
    b) Genital tubercle
    c) Genital swelling
    d) Uro-genital orifice
69. Which accessory sex gland/s in male arises as epithelial outgrowth from caudal region of mesonephric duct:
    a) Seminal vesicle
    b) Prostate and seminal vesicle
    c) Seminal vesicle and bulbo-urethral
    d) Prostate, bulbo-urethral and seminal vesicle
70. Which of the following is located ventral to urogenital folds:
    a) Uro-genital fold
    b) Genital tubercle
    c) Genital swelling
    d) Uro-genital orifice
71. Labio-scrotal swellings is another name for:
    a) Uro-genital fold
    b) Genital tubercle
    c) Genital swelling
    d) Uro-genital orifice
72. The sex cords of the gonads develop from:
    a) Par-axial mesoderm
    b) Intermediate mesoderm
    c) Lateral plate
    d) Notochord
73. In sheep, primordial germ cells can be detected in the genital ridge by:
    a) Day 18
    b) Day 28
    c) Day 22
    d) Day 5

74. In pig, primordial germ cells can be detected in the genital ridge by:
    a) Day 18 b) Day 28
    c) Day 22 d) Day 5

75. In dog, primordial germ cells can be detected in the genital ridge by:
    a) Day 18 b) Day 28
    c) Day 21 d) Day 5

76. In cattle, primordial germ cells can be detected in the genital ridge by:
    a) Day 18 b) Day 28
    c) Day 22 d) Day 5

77. In humans, primordial germ cells can be detected in the genital ridge by:
    a) Day 18 b) Day 28
    c) Day 22 d) Day 5

78. During migration to developing gonads, primordial germ cells undergo:
    a) Mitosis b) Meiosis
    c) Both a & b d) None of the above

79. Appearance of pigment cells in the interstitial tissue during the 9th month of gestation is notable feature of developing testes of:
    a) Equine b) Ruminant
    c) Dog d) Pig

80. In sheep, approximate age when spermatogenesis begins is:
    a) 5 months b) 2 years
    c) 10 months d) 8 months

81. In cattle, approximate age when spermatogenesis begins is:
    a) 5 months b) 2 years
    c) 10 months d) 6-8 months

82. In dog, approximate age when spermatogenesis begins is:
    a) 5 months b) 2 years
    c) 9-10 months d) 8 months

83. In horse, approximate age when spermatogenesis begins is:
    a) 5 months b) 2 years
    c) 10 months d) 8 months

84. Mesenchymal cells under the coelomic epithelium of the developing testis develop into a fibrous layer known as:
    a) Tunica vaginalis b) Tunica albugenia
    c) Rete testis d) Mediastinum testis

85. Mesenchymal cells surrounding the tubules of the rete testis form a fibrous network known as:
    a) Tunica vaginalis b) Tunica albugenia
    c) Mediastinum testis d) Interstitial cells

86. Small vestige of the mesonephric duct cranial to developing testes is known as:
a) Appendix epididymis b) Epoophoron
c) Paroophoron d) Paradidymis

87. Some of the mesonephric tubules at the caudal pole of the developing testes do not join the tubules of the rete testis and gradually lose contact with the mesonephric duct. These vestiges are collectively referred to as:
a) Appendix epididymis b) Epoophoron
c) Paroophoron d) Paradidymis

88. Term 'prostatic utricle' is associated with:
a) Appendix epididymis b) Appendix testis
c) Uterus musculinus d) Paradidymis

89. Os penis is seen in:
a) Goat b) Bull
c) Dog d) Pig

90. Position of scrotum is ventral to anus in:
a) Dog b) Pig
c) Cat d) Both b & c

91. Body of penis develops from:
a) Genital tubercle b) Genital swelling
c) Urogenital fold d) Urogenital sinus

92. Which of the following does not derive from sex cords:
a) Seminiferous tubules b) Sertoli cells
c) Leydig cells d) Spermatozoa

93. Congenital defect in males due to partial failure of the urogenital folds to close in which urethra opens into ventral surface of penis:
a) Penile hypoplasia b) Hypospadias
c) Congenital preputial stenosis d) Persistent penile frenulum

94. Congenital defect in males where urethra opens onto the dorsal surface of a shortened penis is:
a) Penile hypoplasia b) Hypospadias
c) Congenital preputial stenosis d) Epispadia

95. Failure of the normal separation of the glans penis from the preputial epithelium, results in an inability to protrude the penis:
a) Penile hypoplasia b) Hypospadias
c) Congenital preputial stenosis d) Persistent penile frenulum

96. Testes remain within abdominal cavity in:
a) Elephant b) Aquatic mammals
c) Platypus d) All of the above

97. Müllerian inhibiting substance (MIS) is produced by:
   a) Leydig cells b) Graafian follicle
   c) Sertoli cells d) Myoid cells

98. Which of the following structures derive from genital tubercle mesenchyme:
   a) Corpus cavernosum penis, tunica albuginea and corpus spongiosum penis
   b) Tunica albuginea and scrotum
   c) Only scrotum
   d) Scrotum and prepuce

99. Which of the following does not derive from mesonephric duct:
   a) Epididymis b) Vesicular gland
   c) Ductus deferens d) Penile urethra

100. The definitive urogenital sinus forms:
   a) Pelvic urethra b) Penile urethra
   c) Both a & b d) None of the above

101. First critical stage of sexual differentiation occurs at:
   a) Fertilization b) Ovulation
   c) Implantation d) None of the above

102. Sex determining function of Y chromosome is bound with activity of:
   a) Y linked histo-compatibility antigen b) H-Y antigen
   c) Y antigen only d) All of the above

103. Transformation of gonad into testis and ovary completes which stage of sexual differentiation:
   a) 1st b) 2nd
   c) 3rd d) 4th

104. Differentiation of major glands associated with ducts (Prostate and seminal vesicle) depends on:
   a) H-Y antigen b) Androgens
   c) Testosterone d) All of the above

105. In females, which of the following is not secreted by gonads:
   a) Testosterone b) H-Y antigen
   c) Mullerian inhibitory factor d) All of the above

106. Turner's syndrome occurs in which condition:
   a) XXO b) XO
   c) YO d) None of the above

107. In absence of modifying influences, the body has tendency to develop into:
   a) Female line b) Male line
   c) Transgender d) None of the above

108. Final stage of sexual differentiation occurs at the time of:
   a) Fertilization b) Implantation
   c) At birth d) Puberty

109. In hetero-sexual pair of twin cattle, male develop normally and female has characters of male. This condition is known as:

a) Turner's syndrome b) Cushing syndrome

c) Free martin d) None of the above

110. Prostate and cowper's gland develop from ___________ under the influence of testosterone:

a) Urethral epithelium b) Uro-genital sinus (lower)

c) Uro-genital sinus (upper) d) None of the above

Answer Key

1	b	2	a	3	b	4	a	5	a	6	c	7	b
8	c	9	b	10	c	11	d	12	a	13	c	14	a
15	b	16	a	17	b	18	a	19	c	20	d	21	d
22	c	23	d	24	c	25	d	26	c	27	d	28	a
29	c	30	b	31	b	32	a	33	d	34	a	35	b
36	d	37	b	38	a	39	d	40	a	41	b	42	b
43	a	44	b	45	a	46	a	47	b	48	c	49	b
50	c	51	c	52	c	53	c	54	b	55	a	56	b
57	b	58	b	59	a	60	a	61	b	62	d	63	b
64	b	65	b	66	b	67	b	68	c	69	a	70	b
71	c	72	b	73	c	74	a	75	c	76	b	77	b
78	a	79	a	80	a	81	d	82	c	83	b	84	b
85	c	86	a	87	d	88	c	89	c	90	d	91	a
92	d	93	b	94	d	95	d	96	d	97	c	98	a
99	d	100	c	101	a	102	b	103	b	104	c	105	d
106	b	107	a	108	d	109	c	110	a				

21

Development of Integumentary System

Avnish Kumar Gautam, Sanjay Kumar Bharti, Nirbhay Kumar Singh, Manoj Kumar Sinha, Ratnesh Kumar Choudhary and Manoj Kumar Singh

Department of Veterinary Anatomy, Bihar Veterinary College, Bihar Animal Sciences University, Patna, Biar

Introduction

The integumentary system is a vital organ system in animals, encompassing the skin, hair, nails, and associated glands. This complex system is essential for protecting the body, regulating temperature, providing sensory information, and facilitating communication among individuals. The development of the integumentary system is a remarkable evolutionary adaptation that reflects the diverse environmental challenges faced by different species.

The integumentary system has evolved to meet the specific needs of various species, playing a crucial role in survival. As organisms transitioned from aquatic to terrestrial environments, the integument had to adapt to prevent dehydration, protect against UV radiation, and manage temperature fluctuations. For example, the development of a thicker, keratinized epidermis in terrestrial animals minimizes water loss and provides a barrier against environmental stressors.

In mammals, the integumentary system exhibits even greater complexity. The evolution of hair, fur, and other adaptations allows for enhanced thermoregulation, sensory perception, and social interaction. For instance, many mammals have evolved specialized hair types, such as the insulating undercoat found in Arctic species or the short, coarse hair of desert-dwelling animals that aids in heat dissipation.

Anatomical Structure

The integumentary system is composed of several key components: the epidermis, dermis, hypodermis (subcutaneous layer), and associated appendages such as hair follicles, sebaceous glands, and sweat glands.

1. **Epidermis**: The outermost layer of the skin, the epidermis, is primarily composed of keratinocytes, which produce keratin, a protein that provides strength and waterproofing. Melanocytes, located within the epidermis, produce melanin, the pigment responsible for skin color. The thickness of the epidermis varies significantly among species, with adaptations reflecting the ecological niches of each animal.

2. **Dermis**: Beneath the epidermis lies the dermis, which is significantly thicker and contains connective tissue, blood vessels, nerves, and various structures such as hair follicles and glands. The dermis is responsible for providing structural support and elasticity to the skin. It also contains collagen and elastin fibers, which contribute to the skin's resilience.
3. **Hypodermis**: The hypodermis, or subcutaneous layer, is composed of loose connective tissue and fat, which serves as insulation and energy storage. This layer plays a critical role in thermoregulation and helps anchor the skin to underlying structures.
4. **Glands and Appendages**: The integumentary system includes several specialized structures, such as sebaceous glands that produce oils to keep the skin and hair lubricated, and sweat glands that aid in thermoregulation. Hair follicles produce hair, which can serve various functions, including insulation, camouflage, and sensory input.

Developmental Processes

The development of the integumentary system begins early in embryonic life. The skin originates from the ectoderm, which forms the epidermis, while the underlying mesoderm gives rise to the dermis. During the embryonic stage, various signaling pathways guide the differentiation of skin cells, leading to the formation of specialized structures.

1. **Embryonic Development**: The initial stages of skin development involve the proliferation and differentiation of ectodermal cells. The interaction between ectodermal and mesodermal tissues is crucial for proper integument formation. For example, the formation of hair follicles requires signals from the dermal layer to induce the overlying epidermis to form the hair shaft.
2. **Neonatal Development**: As animals are born, their integument continues to mature. Neonatal skin is often thinner and more sensitive than that of adults, making it susceptible to environmental factors. In this stage, the skin undergoes rapid changes, including increased thickness and the establishment of a protective barrier.
3. **Adolescent and Adult Development**: During adolescence, the integument undergoes significant changes influenced by hormonal fluctuations. In many mammals, increased levels of hormones such as testosterone and estrogen lead to changes in hair growth patterns and skin oiliness. In adults, the skin continues to adapt to environmental challenges, with ongoing processes of repair and regeneration.

Overall the development of the integumentary system in animals is a complex and dynamic process shaped by evolutionary pressures, environmental factors, and physiological needs. As a critical interface between the organism and its environment, the integumentary system plays multifaceted roles in protection, regulation, sensation, and communication. Understanding the intricacies of this system not only enhances our knowledge of animal biology but also informs practices in veterinary medicine, conservation, and animal husbandry. By studying the evolution and development of the integumentary system across different species, we gain insights into the remarkable adaptability of life on Earth.

Multiple Choice Questions

1. What is the primary function of the integumentary system in domestic animals?
   a) Digestion b) Sensory perception
   c) Thermoregulation d) Reproduction
2. At what stage of embryonic development does the integumentary system begin to form in mammals?
   a) Blastocyst stage b) Gastrulation
   c) Organogenesis d) Fetal stage
3. The epidermis in domestic animals primarily originates from which embryonic layer?
   a) Endoderm b) Mesoderm
   c) Ectoderm d) Epiblast
4. In which layer of the epidermis does keratinization predominantly occur?
   a) Stratumbasale b) Stratum spinosum
   c) Stratum granulosum d) Stratum corneum
5. What is the primary role of the dermis in the integumentary system?
   a) Structural support and nourishment to the epidermis
   b) Act as a barrier against pathogens
   c) To produce pigment
   d) To regulate body temperature
6. Which type of gland is responsible for the production of sweat in domestic imals?
   a) Sebaceous gland b) Apocrine gland
   c) Exocrinegland d) Mammary gland
7. Which layer of the skin contains hair follicles, sebaceous glands, and sweat glands?
   a) Epidermis b) Hypodermis
   c) Dermis d) Subcutis
8. What is the primary function of sebaceous glands in domestic animals?
   a) To produce hormones b) To secrete sweat
   c) To lubricate and waterproof the skin d) To regulate body temperature
9. What type of hair is primarily responsible for insulation in domestic animals?
   a) Guard hairs b) Undercoat
   c) Vibrissae d) Secondary hairs
10. What is the role of melanocytes in the integumentary system?
    a) To produce keratin b) To provide structural support
    c) To produce pigment d) To secrete sweat
11. During which phase of hair growth does the hair follicle remain dormant?
    a) Anagen b) Catagen
    c) Telogen d) Exogen

12. In which layer of the skin are blood vessels and nerves primarily located?
    a) Epidermis b) Dermis
    c) Hypodermis d) Subcutis
13. What is the name of the condition characterized by excessive shedding or loss of hair in domestic animals?
    a) Alopecia b) Dermatitis
    c) Eczema d) Psoriasis
14. Which type of connective tissue is most commonly found in the dermis of domestic animals?
    a) Adipose tissue b) Dense irregular connective tissue
    c) Loose connective tissue d) Cartilage
15. What structure in the skin helps to sense light touch in domestic animals?
    a) Pacinian corpuscles b) Meissner'scorpuscles
    c) Ruffini endings d) Merkel cells
16. What is the primary component of the extracellular matrix in the dermis?
    a) Collagen b) Elastin
    c) Hyaluronic acid d) Keratin
17. Which domestic animal is known for having a specialized structure called the "dewclaw"?
    a) Horse b) Dog
    c) Cat d) Cow
18. In which domestic animal is the development of the integumentary system most pronounced at birth, with a significant amount of hair or wool?
    a) Pig b) Cow
    c) Sheep d) Chicken
19. What is the primary purpose of the hypodermis in the integumentary system?
    a) To provide a barrier to pathogens b) To cushion and insulate the body
    c) To produce skin cells d) To secrete hormones
20. Which of the following is NOT a function of the integumentary system?
    a) Sensory reception
    b) Production of blood cells
    c) Thermoregulation
    d) Protection from environmental damage
21. Dermis is developed in
    a) Early embryonicperiod b) Late embryonic period
    c) Both d) None
22. Which of the following region does not have hypodermis.
    a) Lip b) Eyelids
    c) Pinna d) All

23. Which of the following cells are act as antigen presenting cells in skin.
a) Langerhans cells b) Merkel cells
c) Melanoblast d) None

24. Melanoblast are derived from
a) Neural crest b) Yolk sac
c) Both d) None

25. The primordial structure of the hair project into the underlying mesoderm to form-
a) Hair buds b) Pegs
c) Both d) None

26. Which of the following structures are the modified cutaneous structures?
a) Horn b) Hoof
c) Beak d) All

27. The first indication of the feather development occurs in a chick embryo at
a) Dayone of development b) 8th day of development
c) 13th day of development d) 20th day of development

28. What germ layer primarily gives rise to the skin?
a) Ectoderm b) Mesoderm
c) Endoderm d) All of the above

29. The outermost layer of the skin is known as the:
a) Dermis b) Epidermis
c) Hypodermis d) Basement membrane

30. Which structure is responsible for the formation of hair follicles?
a) Epidermal ridges b) Dermal papillae
c) Mesenchyme d) Neural crest cells

31. The process by which the epidermis forms is called:
a) Neurulation b) Organogenesis
c) Ectodermal differentiation d) Morphogenesis

32. Which of the following skin appendages develops from the ectoderm?
a) Sweat glands b) Hair follicles
c) Sebaceous glands d) All of the above

33. At what embryonic stage does the skin begin to differentiate?
a) Blastula b) Gastrula
c) Neurula d) Somite stage

34. The development of melanocytes originates from which embryonic structure?
a) Ectoderm b) Mesoderm
c) Neural crest d) Endoderm

35. Which protein is primarily responsible for the structural integrity of the epidermis?
a) Collagen b) Keratin
c) Elastin d) Fibronectin

36. In amphibians, the skin becomes impermeable to water during:
    a) Larval stage b) Metamorphosis
    c) Adult stage d) Fertilization
37. What is the primary function of the epidermis?
    a) Sensation b) Protection
    c) Temperature regulation d) All of the above
38. In reptiles, the skin is primarily characterized by:
    a) Glandular structures b) Scales
    c) Hair follicles d) Feathers
39. The embryonic origin of dermal connective tissue is primarily:
    a) Mesoderm b) Endoderm
    c) Ectoderm d) Neuroectoderm
40. The dermis is primarily made up of:
    a) Stratified squamous epithelium b) Loose connective tissue
    c) Dense irregular connective tissue d) Adipose tissue
41. Which type of skin cell is responsible for the immune response in the epidermis?
    a) Keratinocytes b) Melanocytes
    c) Langerhans cells d) Merkel cells
42. The transition of epidermal cells into a keratinized state is known as:
    a) Apoptosis b) Keratinization
    c) Differentiation d) Proliferation
43. Which factor is crucial for the development of skin appendages?
    a) Sonic hedgehog b) Bone morphogenetic proteins
    c) Fibroblast growth factors d) All of the above
44. The presence of scales in fish is primarily due to:
    a) Dermal origin b) Epidermal origin
    c) Both dermal and epidermal d) Neural crest origin
45. In mammals, which layer of skin contains blood vessels and nerves?
    a) Epidermis b) Dermis
    c) Hypodermis d) All layers
46. The embryological development of feathers is influenced by which signaling pathway?
    a) Wnt b) Notch
    c) Hedgehog d) BMP
47. The process of skin regeneration in amphibians involves:
    a) Cell division only b) Dedifferentiation
    c) Scar formation d) None of the above
48. Which of the following skin structures is not derived from the ectoderm?
    a) Hair b) Nails
    c) Dermis d) Sweat glands

49. Which embryonic layer forms the epidermal layer in mammals?
   a) Ectoderm b) Mesoderm
   c) Endoderm d) All layers
50. In humans, the initial formation of the skin occurs around which week of gestation?
   a) Week 3 b) Week 6
   c) Week 10 d) Week 12
51. In reptiles, the skin is primarily adapted for:
   a) Water absorption b) Thermoregulation
   c) Protection against desiccation d) Sensory perception
52. Which type of cell is responsible for the production of melanin?
   a) Langerhans cells b) Keratinocytes
   c) Melanocytes d) Merkel cells
53. Which layer of the epidermis is responsible for cell division?
   a) Stratum corneum b) Stratum lucidum
   c) Stratum granulosum d) Stratum basale
54. What is the role of the basement membrane in skin development?
   a) Provides structural support b) Regulates cell signaling
   c) Allows nutrient diffusion d) All of the above
55. The embryonic structure that gives rise to the dermal layer of skin is:
   a) Somites b) Neural tube
   c) Lateral plate mesoderm d) All of the above
56. Which protein is abundant in the stratum corneum?
   a) Elastin b) Collagen
   c) Keratin d) Fibronectin
57. Which of the following structures is primarily responsible for thermoregulation in mammals?
   a) Hair follicles b) Sweat glands
   c) Sebaceous glands d) All of the above
58. What is the primary role of sebaceous glands?
   a) Produce sweat b) Provide lubrication to the skin
   c) Produce melanin d) None of the above
59. In which animal group is the skin primarily adapted for gas exchange?
   a) Mammals b) Birds
   c) Amphibians d) Reptiles
60. The outermost layer of fish skin is composed of:
   a) Epidermis b) Scales
   c) Dermis d) Both A and B
61. The embryonic development of nails is similar to that of:
   a) Hair b) Scales
   c) Feathers d) Glands

62. What is the primary function of Merkel cells in the skin?
   a) Sensory perception
   b) Melanin production
   c) Immune response
   d) Keratin production
63. Which embryonic signaling pathway is crucial for the development of hair follicles?
   a) Notch signaling
   b) Wnt signaling
   c) Hedgehog signaling
   d) TGF-beta signaling
64. In mammals, the hypodermis primarily functions as:
   a) Protective barrier
   b) Insulation and energy storage
   c) Sensory reception
   d) Water regulation
65. The condition of skin at the larval stage of amphibians is typically:
   a) Thick and scaly
   b) Thin and permeable
   c) Hairy
   d) Feathered
66. Which type of cell helps to form the waterproof barrier of the skin?
   a) Langerhans cells
   b) Keratinocytes
   c) Melanocytes
   d) Merkel cells
67. In which stage does skin patterning (e.g., scales, feathers) begin to occur?
   a) Cleavage stage
   b) Gastrulation
   c) Organogenesis
   d) Morphogenesis
68. What role does the dermal papillae play in skin?
   a) Sensory function
   b) Nutrient supply to the epidermis
   c) Both A and B
   d) None of the above
69. Which layer of epidermis contains melanocytes.
   a) Stratum corneum
   b) Stratum lucidum
   c) Stratum granulosum
   d) Stratum basale
70. Which fibrous protein is responsible for the strength and water resistance of the skin surface?
   a) Keratohyalin
   b) Eleidin
   c) Collagen
   d) Keratin

Answer Key

1	c	2	c	3	c	4	d	5	a	6	c	7	c
8	c	9	b	10	c	11	c	12	b	13	a	14	b
15	b	16	a	17	d	18	c	19	b	20	b	21	b
22	d	23	a	24	a	25	c	26	d	27	b	28	a
29	b	30	a	31	c	32	d	33	d	34	c	35	b
36	b	37	d	38	b	39	a	40	c	41	c	42	b
43	d	44	a	45	b	46	a	47	b	48	c	49	a
50	b	51	a	52	c	53	d	54	d	55	d	56	a
57	b	58	b	59	c	60	b	61	a	62	a	63	b
64	b	65	b	66	b	67	d	68	c	69	d	70	d

22

Development of the Head and Neck

***Rupam Sinha*[1] *and Ratnesh Kumar Choudhary*[2]**

Department of Veterinary Anatomy, COVs&AH, DUVASU, Mathura, Uttar Pradesh

Department of Veterinary Anatomy, BVC, BASU, Patna, Bihar

Introduction

The development of the head and neck in embryos involves the formation of two primary sections at the cephalic (head) end) These include:

1. **Neural Portion**: This part consists of the brain, eyes, and internal ears, along with their supportive structures. In early embryonic stages, the neural region is larger and more prominent. Even as the face develops, the neural portion retains a dominant role.
2. **Facial or Visceral Portion**: This section encompasses the upper ends of the alimentary (digestive) and respiratory tracts. As the embryo matures, the nose and jaws undergo differentiation and growth, reducing the initial size difference between the neural and facial portions.

Pharyngeal (Branchial) Arches and Their Role

The formation of the face and neck is closely linked with the development of the **pharyngeal (branchial) arches**. These arches appear as bar-like ridges with intervening grooves on the sides of the embryonic head around the fourth week of gestation. Though similar to the gill arches in fish, these structures in mammals do not develop respiratory functions. Instead, they transform into various permanent structures of the adult face and neck.

- **Formation of Pharyngeal Arches and Grooves**: Five pairs of pharyngeal arches typically develop, separated by four ectodermal grooves known as **pharyngeal grooves**. Underneath these grooves, the pharyngeal endoderm pushes the mesenchyme outward, forming **pharyngeal pouches**.
- **Fusion and Separation of Grooves and Pouches**: The ectoderm and endoderm layers of each groove and pouch meet to form thin plates. In some cases, these plates temporarily open, mimicking the gill slit openings of fish. Failure of these openings to close results in a congenital condition known as **branchial fistula**)
- **Role of Pharyngeal Arches in Facial Formation**: The first pharyngeal arch on each side splits into an **upper maxillary** and **lower mandibular process**, forming the basis of the face. The second and third arches play essential roles in forming neck structures.

Development of the Face

The area just below the bulging forebrain and in front of the first pharyngeal arch pair forms the foundation of the face. Key features include the development of the nose, eyes, and nasal (olfactory) pits.

1. **Formation of the Nose and Primary Facial Structures**
   - The **first pharyngeal arch** divides into the maxillary and mandibular processes.
   - The **frontonasal process** initially covers much of the front of the head) Thickened ectoderm on both sides forms the **olfactory placodes** and **nasal pits.** The mandibular processes join to form the **lower jaw**.
2. **Development of Nasal and Maxillary Structures**
   - Each **olfactory placode** evolves into an **olfactory pit**, bordered by a horseshoe-shaped ridge with two extensions: the **median nasal process** and the **lateral nasal process**.
   - The lower part of each median nasal process expands to form **globular processes**. These processes later unite, and the maxillary and nasal processes fuse, closing the **oculo-nasal sulcus** and forming the eye socket.
3. **Final Formation of Facial Features**
   - The **lateral nasal processes** develop into the sides and wings of the nose.
   - The **maxillary processes** create the cheeks, and the frontonasal process gives rise to the forehead)
   - The **philtrum** is formed by the fusion of the two median nasal (globular) processes, while the **chin** forms from the fusion of the mandibular processes.

Congenital Anomalies

Several developmental anomalies may arise due to disruptions in the fusion or formation of these structures:

1. **Aprosopus**: Complete absence of facial features.
2. **Macrostomus**: Incomplete reduction in the width of the primitive mouth slit.
3. **Microstomus**: Excessive narrowing of the mouth slit.
4. **Astomus**: Complete closure of the mouth slit.
5. **Cleft Mandible**: Incomplete fusion of the mandibular processes.
6. **Oblique Facial Cleft**: Failure of fusion between maxillary and lateral nasal processes.
7. **Branchial Fistula**: Incomplete closure of pharyngeal grooves, resembling gill slits.
8. **Cheiloschisis (Harelip)**: Incomplete fusion of the median nasal and maxillary processes, which may be unilateral or bilateral.

Multiple Choice Questions

1. The cellular totipotency was first shown in which domestic animals.

   a) Sheep   b) Dog

   c) Rabbit   d) Horse

2. In cattle placentation is initiated on
   a) 12th day of gestation
   b) 19th day of gestation
   c) 30th day of gestation
   d) 25th day of gestation
3. In cattle first pair of somite is appears on
   a) 12th day of gestation
   b) 19th day of gestation
   c) 20th day of gestation
   d) 25th day of gestation
4. First pair of somite is appearing in sheep on
   a) 12th day of gestation
   b) 19th day of gestation
   c) 15th day of gestation
   d) 25th day of gestation
5. Mesenchyme derived from-----------for the formation of the head region.
   a) Ectodermal placodes
   b) Endodermal placodes
   c) Mesoderm and Ectodermal placodes
   d) Neural crest
6. First functional system develops in embryo is
   a) Cardio-vascular system
   b) Digestive system
   c) Respiratory system
   d) Nervous system
7. Which of the following branch deals with the study of development of animals?
   a) Embryology
   b) Histology
   c) Neurology
   d) Osteology
8. Following is reason for abnormal chromosome numbers in spermatozoa?
   a) Differentiation
   b) Disjunction
   c) Mitosis
   d) Non-disjunction
9. During which of the following exchange of genetic material is takes place?
   a) Cleavage
   b) Meiosis -I
   c) Meiosis-II
   d) Mitosis
10. Which of the following suffixes implies "growth" or "formation"?
   a) Blast
   b) Lemma
   c) Stasis
   d) Cyte
11. Endochondral and intramembranous are two mechanisms of
   a) Bone remodelling
   c) Embryonic skeletal ossification
   b) Controlling blood calcium levels
   d) Cartilage synthesis
12. Pituitary gland is originated from
   a) Ectoderm
   b) Endoderm
   c) Mesoderm
   d) All of the above
13. Thyroid gland is originated from
   a) Ectoderm
   b) Endoderm
   c) Mesoderm
   d) All of the above
14. Restricted development of eye is called as
   a) Nanopthalmia
   b) Exopthalmia
   c) Megolopthalmos
   d) Strabismus

15. Rathke's pouch is the primordium associated with the development of

a) Tongue b) Tooth
c) Pituitary gland d) Stomach

16. Development of face Includes development of orbital, nasal & oral regions, formation, fusion & patterning of .... facial primordia)

a) 5 b) 6
c) 7 d) 8

17. Primordia, proliferation of underlying neural crest derived mesenchyme, include ....fronto-nasal prominence & .... maxillary & mandibular prominences.

a) Single and single b) Single and paired
c) Paired and paired d) Paired and single

18. during development of face .... maxillary prominences merge with fronto-nasal prominence dorsal to stomodeum.

a) Single b) Paired
c) Triple d) None of the above

19. during development of face .... mandibular prominences merge ventral to stomodeum.

a) Single b) Paired
c) Triple d) None of the above

20 . Fronto-nasal prominence, in region of telencephalic bulges, forms 2 sets of bilateral ectodermal thickenings known as ....

a) Nasal placode b) Lens placode
c) Both of the above d) None of the above

21. Nasal placodes, primordia of nasal cavities develop medially on fronto-nasal prominence & located dorsal to maxillary prominences of

a) 1st pharyngeal arches c) 2nd pharyngeal arches
b) 3rd pharyngeal arches d) 4th pharyngeal arches.

22. Lens placodes, develop before the formation of...................placodes, positioned lateral to fronto-nasal primordia)

a) Nasal placode b) Frontal placode
c) Both d) None of the above

23. Mesenchymal proliferations at margins of nasal placodes result in ....shaped medial & lateral nasal prominences.

a) Horse shoe b) Kidney
c) Almond d) Grapes

24. which placodes occupy depressions, by which a process of invagination deepens forming nasal pits.

a) Nasal b) Frontal
c) Maxillary d) Mandibular

25. In carnivores, sheep, goats during development of face the line of fusion is marked by medial groove known as ....

a) Philtrum b) Tongue
c) Placode d) None of the above

26 . which part of the face develops from floor of primordial pharynx.

a) Teeth b) Tongue
c) Eyes d) Ear

27. 3 elevations occur at the level of 1st pharyngeal arch, i.e 2 lateral lingual swellings & a medial swelling is known as ?

a) Tuberculum impar b) Philtrum
c) Lyssa d) None of the above

28. An elevation in the region of second pharyngeal arch is called as

a) Uvula b) Copula
c) Nobula d) None of the above

29. An eminence in the region of third and fourth arch is called as

a) Hypopharyngeal eminence b) Epipharyngeal eminence
b) Both of the above d) None of the above

30. In cattle, the ....swelling contributes to the formation of torus linguae.

a) Medial lingual b) Lateral lingual
c) Middle lingual d) None of the above

31. In .... the line of fusion of lateral swellings can be recognized as median groove.

a) Cattle b) Pig
c) Dog d) Fowl

32. The epithelium of the anterior two third of tongue is derived from?

a) Ectoderm b) Endoderm
c) Mesoderm d) All of the above

33. The epithelium of the caudal one third part of tongue is derived from?

a) Ectoderm b) Endoderm
c) Mesoderm d) All of the above

34. Towards the end of the embryonic period, lingual papillae develops on the surface of the tongue as epithelial outgrowth induced by underlying ....

a) Ectoderm b) Endoderm
c) Mesoderm d) All of the above

35. .... papillae arise from underlying mesoderm & contain nerve endings sensitive to mechanical pressure.

a) Fungiform b) Filiform
c) Circumvallate d) Foliate

36. .... papillae develop by proliferation of epithelium at boundary of body & root of tongue.
   a) Fungiform b) Filiform
   c) Circumvallate d) Vallate

37. .... papillae are formed from epithelial folding on lateral aspect of root of tongue.
   a) Fungiform b) Filiform
   c) Circumvallate d) Foliate

38. which papillae Absent in ruminants.
   a) Fungiform b) Filiform
   c) Circumvallate d) Foliate

39. Taste bud development is promoted by interaction between epithelial cells of papillae & gustatory neurons of cranial nerves ....
   a) 7th b) 9th
   c) 10th d) all the of the above

40. Taste buds are associated with
   a) fungiform b) vallate
   c) foliate papillae d) all of the above

41. Musculature of tongue derives from ....which migrate from occipita myotomes.
   a) Myoblast b) osteoblast
   c) fibroblast d) all of the above

42. Connective tissue & vasculature of tongue are formed from .... mesenchyme.
   a) Pharyngeal b) brachial
   c) both of the above d) none of the above

43. Abnormally large tongue because of the oversized muscle mass.
   a) Macroglossia b) macroglossia /aglossia
   c) bifid tongu d) trifid tongue

44. condition due to the developmental arrest in the body of the tongue.
   a) Macroglossia b) macroglossia /aglossia
   c) bifid tongue d) trifid tongue

45. Unfused lateral swellings and the tuberculum impar leads to development of...........
   a) Macroglossia b) macroglossia /aglossia
   c) bifid tongue d) trifid tongue

46. The salivary glands develop as solid ingrowths of ....in the oral cavity.
   a) Muscular tissue b) nervous tissue
   c) epithelium d) connective tissue

47. The......................salivary gland probably ectodermal in origin in the labiogingival groove.
   (a) Parotid
   b) mandibular
   c) sublingual
   d) none of the above

48. The epithelium of duct and parenchyma of................salivary gland and.............. salivary gland is endodermal in origin.
   a) Parotid
   b) mandibular
   c) sublingual
   d) both b and c are correct

49. Clusters of .... ingrowths give rise to a number of diffuse minor salivary glands which open into the oral cavity.
   a) Oral epithelial
   b) Orbital epithelial
   c) both of the above
   d) none of the above

50. Teeth develop following interaction of ....of dental lamina and underlying ....derived mesenchyme.
   a) Ectoderm and neural crest
   b) mesoderm and neural crest
   c) endoderm and mesoderm
   d) all of the above

51. As the dental buds extend into the mesenchyme, they become cap shaped (dental cap) with inner and outer layers of epithelial cells with reticular cells called........................
   a) Stellate reticulum
   b) dental reticulum
   c) mesenchymal reticulum
   d) none of the above

52. The epithelial cells of the inner layer differentiate into .... which are responsible for the production of ....
   a) Ameloblast and enamel
   b) odontoblast and dentine
   c) both of the above
   d) none of the above

53. The underlying mesenchymal cells of the dental papilla differentiate into tall columnar cells which form ....responsible for formation of ....
   a) Ameloblast and enamel
   b) odontoblast and dentine
   c) both of the above
   d) none of the above

54. Odontoblasts form predentin at tip of papilla which with deposition of crystals of hydroxyapatite & fluoroapatite get mineralised to form ....
   a) Enamel
   b) Dentin
   c) both of the above
   d) none of the above

55. The bones of the skull develop from.......................which surrounds the developing brain.
   a) Mesenchyme
   b) neural crest cells
   c) osteoblast
   d) all of the above

56. The skull may be considered as consisting of two major subdivisions, the ....which surrounds the brain, and the other is known as ....

a) Neuro-cranium and viscero-cranium

b) Viscero-cranium and neuro-cranium

c) both of the above are correct

d) none of the above

57. ....craniumconstitutessupportivestructuralcomponentsoftheoral cavity, pharynx and upper respiratory system.

a) Neuro
b) Viscero
c) both of the above
d) none of the above

58. ....resultsfromthefailureoffusionbetweenthemaxillaryandmedialnasal prominences. It is often associated with cleft palate.

a) Cleft palate
b) cleft lip
c) both of the above
d) none of the above

59. ....is incomplete fusion of the fronto-nasal prominence with the maxillary prominence.

a) Cleft palate
b) cleft lip
c) both of the above
d) none of the above

60. Developmental failure of mandible

a) Agnathia
b) Brachygnathia
c) both of the above
d) none of the above

61. Mandibleismarkedlyshorterthanthemaxillaandthisconditioniscommonlyreferredas overgrowth jaw or parrot mouth.

a) Agnathia
b) Brachygnathia
c) both of the above
d) none of the above

62. Mandible is longer than the maxilla This condition is normal in brachycephalic dogs and Persian cats.

a) Agnathia
b) Brachygnathia
c) prognathia
d) none of the above

63. Failure in the development of the caudal opening between the nasal cavity and pharynx.

a) Choanal stenosis
b) choanal atresia
c) both of the above
d) none of the above

64. ....condition in pups develop due to the failure of lateral lingual processes to develop and the formation of tongue solely from the medial lingual swelling results in small pointed tongue like chicken's tongue.

a) Bird tongue
b) Bird Lip
c) Bird Eye
d) Bird beak

65. ....cysts due to failure of 2nd pharyngeal arch to overgrow the 2nd and 3rd pharyngeal clefts results in cyst like structures found subcutaneously in the pharyngeal region.

a) Pharyngeal crest
b) brachial crest
c) pharyngeal pouch
d) brachial pouch

66. Both eyes are derived from a single field of the .... plate.

a) Neural plate
b) muscular crest
c) neural crest cells
d) ectodermal plate

67. Ectomesenchyme (from neural crest) surrounding the optic cup condenses to form inner and outer layers, the future.......................respectively.

a) Choroid and sclera
b) cornea and sclera
c) ciliary body and choroid
d) optic lens and optic placode

68. The eyelids are formed by upper and lower folds of ....

a) Ectoderm
b) Mesoderm
c) Endoderm
d) none of the above

69 An ....develops in surface ectoderm adjacent to the hindbrain.

a) Optic placode
b) Otic placode
c) both
d) none of the above

70. Otic placode invaginates to form a cup which then closes and separates from the ectoderm, forming an .... and ....

a) Otic cyst and otic capsule
b) otocyst and optic capsule
c) otic vesicle and optic vesicle
d) otic capsule and optic capsule

71. Along its length, the endoderm of esophagus is surrounded by somatic mesoderm of head which develops into ....

a) Smooth muscle
b) striated muscle
c) both types of muscle
d) none of the above

72. The respiratory primordium develops as a ventral groove in the floor of the foregut at the level of -----------------------pharyngeal arch.

a) 2nd
b) 4th
c) 3rd
d) 5th

73. The epithelium of larynx is derived from ....

a) Foregut endoderm
b) midgut ectoderm
c) hindgut ectoderm
d) foregut mesoderm

74. A single swelling develops from the mesoderm of left and right third pharyngeal arches give rise to ....

a) Thyroid cartilage
b) epiglottid cartilage
c) cricoid cartilage
d) aretenoid cartilage

75. .... of both oral and neural origin contributes to the formation of the pituitary gland (hypophysis cerebri).

a) Ectoderm
b) mesoderm
c) endoderm
d) all of the above

76. That portion of the pituitary gland which develops from an upward evagination of oral ectoderm is referred to as the

a) Adenohypophysis b) Neurohypophysis

c) Intermediate Part d) all of the above

77 . The primordial structure from which the adenohypophysis develops is known as ....

a) Adenohypophysis b) Neurohypophysis

c) Intermediate Part d) Rathek's Pouch

78. Asecondcomponentofthepituitarygland,theneurohypophysis,developsfromaventral diverticulum in the floor of the diencephalon known as the ....

a) Adenohypophysis b) Neurohypophysis

c) Infundibulum d) Rathek's Pouch

79. The.........................gland developsas a dorsal neuro-epithelial diverticulum of the caudal part of the roof of the diencephalon.

a) Pituitary b) Pineal

c) Thyroid d) Parathyroid

80. The neuro-epithelial cells of.........................gland differentiate into pinealocytes and glial cells.

a) Pituitary b) pineal

c) thyroid d) parathyroid

81. The...........................gland develops as a ventral midline endodermal diverticulum from the floor of the foregut at a level between the first and second pharyngeal arches.

a) Pituitary b) Pineal

c) Thyroid d) Parathyroid

82. Theparathyroidglandsdevelopfromthedorsalsegmentsofthe...........and............ pharyngeal pouches.

a) 3rd and 4th b) 2nd and 3rd

c) 2nd and 4th d) 4th and 5th

83. The.........................cells are derived from the caudal part of 4th pouch (ultimobrachial body) of the brachial appratus.

a) Pineal cells b) parafollicular

c) follicular d) Piuicytes

84. The.........................is a small gland found in neck region (in many sps) develop from 4th pharyngeal pouch and will give rise to 'C' cell/parafollicular cells.

a) ultimobrachial body b) ultimobrachial gland

c) both of the above d) none of the above

85. The......................... develops from the ventral portion of the left and right third pharyngeal pouches, with a minor contribution in some species from the fourth pharyngeal pouches.

a) Thyroid
b) parathyroid
c) Thymus
d) pituitary

86. ....may occur due to presence of anti-thyroid antibody in mother. It leadsto cretinism.

a) Agenesis of thyroid
b) hypergenesis of thyroid
c) none of the above
d) all of the above

87. .... it develops due to failure of the thyroglossal duct to grow downward and the thyroid gland develops within the tongue.

a) Agenesis of thyroid
b) hypergenesis of thyroid
c) Lingual thyroid
d) all of the above

88. Smallmassesofthyroidtissuehavebeenfoundtobegrowninlarynx,trachea,esophagus, pleura etc called as

a) Agenesis of thyroid
b) hypergenesis of thyroid
c) Ectopic thyroid
d) all of the above

89. Towards the end of the ....week of embryological development.

a) 3rd
b) 4th
c) 5th
d) 6th

90. Due to the failure of neural tube closure, induction of overlying vertebral arches is disruptedIf the arches failtofuse along the dorsal midline, the resulting open vertebral canal is known as

a) Spina bifida
b) spina unifida
c) spina trifida
d) all of the above

91. Complete failure of the neural tube to close is called as .... which is fatal.

a) Rachischisis
b) Spina bifida
c) both of the above
d) none of the above

92 . Duetospinabifidainvolvingmorethantwovertebraethemeningesisinclinedtoherniate results in subcutaneous bulge called as ....

a) Rachischisis
b) spina bifida
c) meningocaele
d) none of the above

93. Thecranialexpandedregionofneuralplategivesrisetodilatationscalledprimarybrain vesicles

a) Prosencephalon (forebrain)
b) Mesencephalon (midbrain),
b) Rhombencephalon (hind brain
d) all of the above

94. Mesencephalon give rise to

a) corpora quadrigemina
b) tegmentum, red nucleus
c) substantia nigra
d) all of the above

95 The rhombencephalon forms dilatations as

a) metencephalon
b) myelencephalon with dilated lumina
c) both of the above
d) none of the above

96\. The myelencephalon gives rise to........................ and it contains nuclei for cranial nerves 5th, 6th,7th,8th,9th,10th,12th.

a) Cerebellum
b) medulla oblongata
c) brain stem
d) all of the above

97 A large cranial defect leads to herniation of meninges and part of brain and is called as---------

a) Encepahlocoele
b) megalocoele
c) microcephalocoele
d) all of the above

98 Asinglecentrallylocatedorbitwhichcontainsanormaleyeorrudimentaryeyeortwoeyes with different degrees of fusion called as

a) Singlopia
b) cyclopia
c) biopia
d) myopia

99 Accumulations of excessive amounts of CSF in the cranial cavity.

a) Hydrocephalous
b) microcepahous
c) both of the above
d) none of the above

100 A condition in which herniation of cerebellar tissue occurs through foramen magnum.

a) Arnold-chiari malformation
b) cyclopia
c) myopia
d) hydrocephalous

Answer Key

1	a	2	b	3	c	4	c	5	c	6	d	7	a
8	d	9	b	10	a	11	c	12	a	13	b	14	a
15	c	16	a	17	b	18	b	19	b	20	c	21	a
22	a	23		24	a	25	c	26	b	27	a	28	b
29	a	30	a	31	c	32	a	33	b	34	c	35	b
36	d	37	d	38	d	39	d	40	d	41	a	42	a
43	a	44	c	45	d	46	c	47	a	48	a	49	a
50		51	a	52	a	53	b	54	b	55	a	56	a
57	c	58	b	59	a	60	a	61	b	62	c	63	c
64	b	65	a	66	a	67	a	68	a	69	b	70	a
71	c	72	b	73	a	74	b	75	a	76	a	77	d
78	c	79	b	80	b	81	c	82	a	83	b	84	c
85	c	86	a	87	c	88	c	89	a	90	a	91	a
92	c	93	d	94	d	95	d	96	b	97	a	98	b
99	a	100	a										

23

Development of Endocrine System

Tolly Bora[1], Anindita Sandilya[1], Monalisha Debbarma[2] and Mohamed Hasif Ganimattoullah[3]

[1]*College of Veterinary sciences and Animal Husbandry, Selesih, Aizawl, Mizoram*

[2]*Department of Veterinary Anatomy and Histology, Institute of Veterinary Science and Animal Husbandry, Siksha O Anusandhan University, Odisha*

[3]*Department of Veterinary Physiology, Institute of vVeterinary Science and Animal Husbandry, Siksha O Anusandhan University, Odisha*

Introduction

The endocrine system consists of glands and cells that secrete hormones directly into surrounding tissues or into the bloodstream to regulate various physiological processes. These hormones help maintain homeostasis, working closely with the nervous system, especially through the hypothalamo-hypophyseal connection, where the endocrine and nervous systems integrate their functions.

Pituitary Gland (Hypophysis)

The pituitary gland, often considered the "master gland," is formed from oral and neural ectoderm. It is divided into two main parts: the anterior pituitary (adenohypophysis) and the posterior pituitary (neurohypophysis).

Adenohypophysis: This portion develops from the roof of the stomodeum (primitive mouth) and consists of three parts: the pars distalis, pars intermedia, and pars tuberalis. It contains several cell types, including acidophils, basophils, and chromophobes, which secrete various hormones. For instance, acidophils release growth hormone (GH) and prolactin, while basophils produce hormones like adrenocorticotropic hormone (ACTH), thyroid-stimulating hormone (TSH), and gonadotropins (LH and FSH). The secretion of these hormones is regulated by the hypothalamus through releasing and inhibitory factors delivered via the hypophyseal portal system.

Neurohypophysis: Originating from the floor of the diencephalon, the neurohypophysis consists of the median eminence, infundibular stalk, and neural lobe. It stores and releases antidiuretic hormone (ADH) and oxytocin, both synthesized in the hypothalamus and transported to the posterior pituitary. ADH regulates water balance, while oxytocin controls uterine contractions and milk ejection during lactation.

Hypothalamo-Hypophyseal System

The hypothalamus and pituitary gland form a unified control system. The hypothalamo-adenohypophyseal system is responsible for regulating the anterior pituitary's hormonal release. Neurosecretory cells in the hypothalamus produce hormones such as growth hormone-releasing hormone (GHRH), gonadotropin-releasing hormone (GnRH), and corticotropin-releasing hormone (CRH). These hormones travel through the hypophyseal portal system to stimulate or inhibit the secretion of corresponding hormones from the anterior pituitary.

In contrast, the hypothalamo-neurohypophyseal system is more straightforward)
Here, hormones like ADH and oxytocin are synthesized in the hypothalamic neurons and transported along axons to be stored in the posterior pituitary until they are released into the bloodstream in response to specific stimuli.

Pineal Gland

The pineal gland is a small endocrine organ located in the roof of the diencephalon. It secretes melatonin, a hormone involved in regulating circadian rhythms, especially sleep-wake cycles, and reproductive functions. Melatonin release is influenced by light exposure; it increases during darkness and decreases in response to daylight. This light-sensitive regulation allows the pineal gland to synchronize biological processes with environmental light cycles. The pineal gland is composed of pinealocytes and is permeated by a network of capillaries, ensuring efficient hormone distribution.

Thymus

The thymus, essential for immune function, develops from the third and fourth pharyngeal pouches. During embryogenesis, it extends caudally, eventually fusing in the midline. The thymus plays a critical role in the maturation of T lymphocytes, which are vital for cell-mediated immunity. Thymocytes within the thymus differentiate into various types of T cells, which then migrate to other lymphoid tissues to carry out immune functions. The thymus is most active during childhood and gradually atrophies after puberty.

Thyroid Gland

The thyroid gland originates from the floor of the foregut and later divides into two lobes connected by an isthmus. Its primary function is to produce thyroid hormones (thyroxine [T4] and triiodothyronine [T3]), which regulate metabolism, growth, and development. The follicular cells of the thyroid gland synthesize these hormones by absorbing iodine from the bloodstream. Thyroid hormone production is controlled by thyroid-stimulating hormone (TSH) from the anterior pituitary. In addition, the gland contains parafollicular cells (C cells) that secrete calcitonin, a hormone that helps regulate calcium levels by reducing blood calcium concentration, opposing the effects of parathyroid hormone (PTH).

Parathyroid Glands

The parathyroid glands develop from the dorsal portions of the third and fourth pharyngeal pouches. These small glands are located near the thyroid gland and play a key role in calcium homeostasis. They secrete parathyroid hormone (PTH), which increases blood calcium levels by promoting calcium absorption in the intestines, reducing calcium excretion in the kidneys, and stimulating calcium release from bones. PTH works in opposition to calcitonin from the thyroid gland to maintain a balanced calcium level necessary for nerve function, muscle contraction, and blood clotting.

Adrenal Glands

The adrenal glands, located atop the kidneys, consist of two distinct parts: the cortex and the medulla, which originate from different embryological tissues. The adrenal cortex is derived from mesoderm and is divided into three zones:

1. **Zona glomerulosa**: Produces mineralocorticoids like aldosterone, which regulate electrolyte and water balance.
2. **Zona fasciculata**: Secretes glucocorticoids such as cortisol, which regulate metabolism and immune responses.
3. **Zona reticularis**: Produces androgens, contributing to secondary sexual characteristics.

The adrenal medulla, derived from neural crest cells, functions as part of the sympathetic nervous system. It secretes epinephrine and norepinephrine in response to stress, preparing the body for the "fight or flight" response by increasing heart rate, blood pressure, and energy availability.

Pancreatic Islets (Islets of Langerhans)

The pancreas has both exocrine and endocrine functions, with its endocrine role centered in the islets of Langerhans, which consist of different cell types:

Alpha (α) cells: Secrete glucagon, which raises blood glucose levels by promoting glycogen breakdown in the liver.

Beta (β) cells: Produce insulin, which lowers blood glucose by facilitating glucose uptake in cells.

Delta (δ) cells: Release somatostatin, which inhibits the secretion of both insulin and glucagon, maintaining balance in glucose metabolism.

These islet cells work together to regulate blood glucose levels, ensuring metabolic stability. Glucagon and insulin have opposing effects, with glucagon increasing and insulin decreasing blood sugar levels. Somatostatin modulates the release of these hormones to prevent extremes in glucose fluctuations.

Multiple Choice Questions

1. The adenohypophysis is also known as which part of the pituitary gland?
   a) Anterior pituitary b) Posterior pituitary
   c) Intermediate lobe d) Hypothalamus
2. Which hormone is NOT produced by the pars distalis?
   a) Growth hormone (STH) b) Prolactin
   c) Melatonin d) Thyrotropin (TSH)
3. What is the function of the hypothalamo-adenohypophyseal system?
   a) To release digestive enzymes
   b) To synthesize and transport hormonesc.
   c) To stimulate the secretion of thyroid hormones
   d) To inhibit the function of the adrenal cortex

4. Which of the following is a hormone that inhibits the release of growth hormone?
   a) Somatotropin b) Somatostatinc
   c) Prolactin d) Thyrotropin
5. Which cells are characterized by having secretory granules that stain with orange G and measure 300 to 400 nm in diameter?
   a) Corticotropes b) Lactotropes
   c) Somatotropes d) Gonadotropes
6. Which of the following cells is most abundant in the pars intermedia of domestic mammals?
   a) Somatotropes b) Melanotropes
   c) Thyrotropes d) Lactotropes
7. Which of the following is the largest type of secretory granule found in the adenohypophysis?
   a) Somatotrope granules b) Lactotrope granule
   c) Gonadotrope granules d) Thyrotrope granules
8. Which of the following cells in the adenohypophysis are known for their strong periodic acid-Schiff (PAS) reaction due to the presence of glycoprotein hormones?
   a) Somatotropes b) Basophils
   c) Lactotropes d) Chromophobes
9. What is the main function of β-endorphin?
   a) Inhibits the release of growth hormone
   b) Promotes the dispersion of melanophores
   c) Acts similarly to morphine, providing pain relief
   d) Stimulates the secretion of glucocorticoids
10. Which structure surrounds the median eminence like a sleeve and contains specific secretory cells involved in seasonal reproduction?
    a) Pars distalis b) Pars intermedia
    c) Pars tuberalis d) Neurohypophysis
11. The neurohypophysis develops as a ventral outgrowth from which part of the brain?
    a) Cerebellum b) Hypothalamus
    c) Thalamus d) Medulla oblongata
12. Which cells are scattered among the epithelium of the gastrointestinal and respiratory systems and have endocrine functions?
    a) Thyrotropes b) Chromophobes
    c) Single cells with endocrine functions d) Somatotropes
13. Which of the following best describes the origin of the adenohypophysis during embryonic development?
    a) Ventral outgrowth of the hypothalamus
    b) Dorsal evagination of the epithelial roof of the embryonic pharynx
    c) Lateral evagination of the neural tube
    d) Outgrowth from the diencephalon

14. The primary capillary plexus of the hypophyseal portal system is located in which region?
    a) Pars distalis
    b) Median eminence
    c) Pars intermedia
    d) Infundibular stalk
15. Where are hypothalamic neurohormones released into the hypophyseal portal system?
    a) Pars distalis
    b) Median eminence
    c) Pars intermedia
    d) Infundibular stalk
16. The main secretory product of pinealocytes is:
    a) Melatonin
    b) Serotonin
    c) Dopamine
    d) Oxytocin
17. What drives the secretion of melatonin?
    a) Light phase of the photoperiod
    b) Dark phase of the photoperiod
    c) Increased plasma osmolality
    d) Mechanical stimulation
18. The main cell type in the parathyroid gland is:
    a) Chief cells
    b) Oxyphil cells
    c) Pinealocytes
    d) Follicular cells
19. The thymus develops primarily from which pharyngeal pouches?
    a) First and second
    b) Second and third
    c) Third and fourth
    d) Fourth and fifth
20. In which species does the embryonic thymus maintain its Y-shaped structure with cranial, cervical, and thoracic regions into the neonatal stage?
    a) Horses
    b) Carnivores
    c) Humans
    d) Ruminants and pigs
21. During thymus development, what do the neural crest-derived mesenchymal cells form?
    a) Thymic or Hassall's corpuscles
    b) A connective tissue capsule
    c) Bone marrow
    d) The cranial mediastinal space
22. What is the primary function of the blood–thymus barrier?
    a) To allow the entry of foreign antigens into the thymus
    b) To produce hormones like thymosin and thymopoietin
    c) To isolate T lymphocytes from antigenic challenge
    d) To facilitate the migration of pro-thymocytes
23. What happens to the thymus with the onset of sexual maturity?
    a) It becomes more prominent
    b) It undergoes gradual involution
    c) It produces more T lymphocytes
    d) It develops additional thymic corpuscles
24. During the early embryonic period, which cells migrate to the developing thymus?
    a) Epithelial cells
    b) Neural crest cells
    c) Pro-thymocytes
    d) Adipocytes

25. Thymic or Hassall's corpuscles are formed by which type of cells?
    a) Bone marrow-derived cells
    b) Neural crest-derived mesenchymal cells
    c) Concentric layers of squamous medullary epithelial cells
    d) Thymocytes
26. Which hormones produced by epithelial reticular cells are crucial for the maturation of pro-thymocytes into T lymphocytes?
    a) Insulin and glucagon
    b) Thymosin and thymopoietin
    c) Estrogen and testosterone
    d) Cortisol and adrenaline
27. In which species does the entire cervical portion of the thymus regress, leaving only the thoracic part as a bilobed structure?
    a) Horses
    b) Pigs
    c) Ruminants
    d) Carnivores and humans
28. What structural change characterizes thymic involution?
    a) Increase in thymocyte numbers
    b) Enlargement of epithelial reticular cells
    c) Formation of additional blood vessels
    d) Expansion of the cortex
29. The thyroid gland develops from which embryonic structure?
    a) Lateral pharyngeal pouches
    b) Ventral midline endodermal diverticulum
    c) Dorsal midline ectodermal tissue
    d) Neural crest cells
30. Where does the thyroid gland initially develop?
    a) Between the second and third pharyngeal arches
    b) Between the third and fourth pharyngeal arches
    c) Between the first and second pharyngeal arches
    d) Between the fourth and fifth pharyngeal arches
31. What structure connects the developing thyroid gland to the foregut initially?
    a) Thyro-pharyngeal duct
    b) Tracheo-glossal duct
    c) Thyro-glossal duct
    d) Pharyngo-tracheal duct
32. During development, the thyroid gland migrates to a position
    a) Lateral to the trachea
    b) Dorsal to the foregut
    c) Ventral to the developing trachea
    d) Posterior to the pharynx
33. What forms the isthmus in the developing thyroid gland?
    a) Neural crest cells
    b) Mesodermal tissue
    c) Glandular tissue connecting the lobes
    d) Pharyngeal arches
34. In which species is the isthmus of the thyroid gland particularly substantial?
    a) Horses and ruminants
    b) Pigs and humans
    c) Carnivores and ruminants
    d) Birds and reptiles

35. Thyroid hormones thyroxine (T4) and tri-iodothyronine (T3) are synthesized by:
    a) Neural crest-derived cells
    b) Cuboidal epithelial cells
    c) Parafollicular cells
    d) Ultimo-branchial body cells
36. Which gland produces thyroid-stimulating hormone (TSH) that regulates thyroid hormone synthesis and release?
    a) Parathyroid gland
    b) Adrenal gland
    c) Pituitary gland (pars distalis)
    d) Hypothalamus
37. Which structure becomes incorporated into the thyroid tissue during its caudal migration?
    a) Dorsal pharyngeal pouches
    b) Ultimo-branchial bodies
    c) Neural tube
    d) Pharyngeal arches
38. What do the cells of the ultimo-branchial body give rise to in the thyroid gland?
    a) Cuboidal epithelial cells
    b) Osteoclasts
    c) C-cells or parafollicular cells
    d) Follicular cells
39. How does calcitonin affect bone metabolism?
    a) Stimulates bone resorption by osteoclasts
    b) Inhibits calcium deposition in bone
    c) Promotes calcium deposition in bone
    d) Stimulates osteoblast activity
40. The thyroid primordium is initially attached to the foregut by which of the following?
    a) Ultimo-branchial body
    b) Thyro-glossal duct
    c) Neural tube
    d) Isthmus
41. The thyroid gland is located on which aspect of the developing trachea?
    a) Dorsal
    b) Ventral
    c) Lateral
    d) Posterior
42. The parathyroid glands develop from which parts of the pharyngeal pouches?
    a) Ventral segments of the third and fourth pharyngeal pouches
    b) Dorsal segments of the second and third pharyngeal pouches
    c) Dorsal segments of the third and fourth pharyngeal pouches
    d) Ventral segments of the first and second pharyngeal pouches
43. The external parathyroid or parathyroid III gland originates from which pharyngeal pouch?
    a) First pharyngeal pouch
    b) Second pharyngeal pouch
    c) Third pharyngeal pouch
    d) Fourth pharyngeal pouch
44. What causes the parathyroid III glands to occupy a position caudal to the parathyroid IV glands?
    a) Thyroid gland migration
    b) Thymus migration
    c) Pharyngeal wall attachment
    d) Neural crest cell migration

45. Where are the parathyroid IV glands typically located in relation to the thyroid gland?
    a) Caudal to the thyroid gland
    b) Lateral to the thyroid gland
    c) Embedded within the thyroid gland
    d) Ventral to the thyroid gland
46. In which species are the parathyroid III glands located close to the thoracic inlet due to thymus migration?
    a) Pigs
    b) Humans
    c) Horses
    d) Ruminants
47. Which parathyroid glands regress in pigs, resulting in only one type developing?
    a) Parathyroid III glands
    b) Parathyroid IV glands
    c) Both parathyroid III and IV glands
    d) Neither parathyroid III nor IV glands
48. What is the primary function of the chief cells in the parathyroid glands?
    a) Secretion of calcitonin
    b) Secretion of parathyroid hormone (parathormone)
    c) Secretion of thyroid hormones
    d) Secretion of adrenaline
49. Parathyroid hormone (PTH) increases blood calcium levels by:
    a) Stimulating osteoclasts to release calcium from bone
    b) Inhibiting calcium absorption from dietary sources
    c) Promoting calcium excretion by the kidneys
    d) Stimulating calcitonin release
50. How does parathyroid hormone affect calcium deposition in bones?
    a) It promotes calcium deposition
    b) It inhibits calcium deposition
    c) It has no effect on calcium deposition
    d) It increases calcitonin secretion to inhibit deposition
51. Which of the following is a function of parathyroid hormone (PTH) in the kidneys?
    a) Promotes calcium excretion
    b) Increases calcium absorption
    c) Decreases calcium excretion
    d) Inhibits calcium absorption
52. The function of oxyphil cells in the parathyroid glands is:
    a) Well-defined and involves hormone secretion
    b) Unknown and undetermined
    c) Related to T3 and T4 production
    d) Involved in the regulation of thyroid hormones
53. Which gland develops from the dorsal segments of the fourth pharyngeal pouches?
    a) Parathyroid III glands
    b) Parathyroid IV glands
    c) Thyroid gland
    d) Thymus

54. What happens to the connection between the parathyroid gland primordia and the pharyngeal wall during development?

a) It strengthens
b) It becomes more complex
c) It remains unchanged
d) It is lost

55. In the final position, where are the parathyroid III glands typically located?

a) Ventral to the thyroid gland
b) Caudal to the thyroid gland
c) Embedded within the thyroid gland
d) Lateral to the thymus

56. Which species has only parathyroid III glands due to the regression of parathyroid IV glands?

a) Horses
b) Pigs
c) Humans
d) Ruminants

57. What effect does parathyroid hormone have on dietary calcium absorption?

a) It inhibits dietary calcium absorption
b) It promotes dietary calcium absorption
c) It has no effect on dietary calcium absorption
d) It decreases dietary calcium absorption

58. How do parathyroid glands differ between most domestic species and pigs?

a) Pigs have both parathyroid III and IV glands
b) Pigs have no parathyroid glands
c) Pigs have only parathyroid III glands
d) Pigs have only parathyroid IV glands

59. Which glands are drawn caudally by the developing thymus during embryonic development?

a) Parathyroid III glands only
b) Parathyroid IV glands only
c) Both parathyroid III and IV glands
d) Neither parathyroid III nor IV glands

60. What do the pancreatic islets, or islets of Langerhans, develop from?

a) Endocrine component of the pancreas
b) Exocrine component of the pancreas
c) Hepatocytes
d) Myocytes

61. Which cells within the pancreatic islets produce insulin?

a) α-cells
b) β-cells
c) δ-cells
d) G cells

62. Which cell type in the pancreatic islets is responsible for secreting pancreatic polypeptide?

a) α-cells
b) β-cells
c) PP cells
d) δ-cells

63. From which embryological tissues do the paired mammalian adrenal glands develop?
   a) Endoderm and ectoderm
   b) Neural crest cell ectoderm and intermediate mesoderm
   c) Mesoderm and endoderm
   d) Neural tube and somites

64. What are the two components of the adrenal gland?
   a) Outer medulla and inner cortex b) Outer cortex and inner medulla
   c) Glomerulosa and reticularis d) Medulla and fasciculate

65. In fish, how are the tissues that correspond to the adrenal gland in mammals organized?
   a) As a single integrated gland b) In direct contact
   c) As two separate endocrine organs d) Randomly integrated

66. What does the neural crest-derived tissue in mammals form?
   a) Adrenal cortex b) Zona glomerulosa
   c) Adrenal medulla d) Mesonephros

67. Which part of the adrenal gland is derived from intermediate mesoderm?
   a) Medulla b) Cortex
   c) Glomerulosa d) Chromaffin cells

68. What is the initial large adrenal cortex called during fetal development?
   a) Definitive cortex b) Fetal cortex
   c) Mesodermal cortex d) Neonatal cortex

69. Which layer of the adrenal cortex produces the mineralocorticoid hormone aldosterone?
   a) Zona glomerulosa b) Zona fasciculata
   c) Zona reticularis d) Zona pellucida

70. What hormone does the fetal adrenal cortex produce at higher levels than the definitive cortex?
   a) Cortisol b) Aldosterone
   c) Steroid hormones d) Epinephrine

71. Which hormone plays a major role in the initiation of parturition in many mammalian species?
   a) Aldosterone b) Epinephrine
   c) Norepinephrine d) Cortisol

72. The adrenal medulla resembles a modified ganglion of which system?
   a) Parasympathetic nervous system b) Enteric nervous system
   c) Sympathetic nervous system d) Central nervous system

73. What stimulates the secretion of epinephrine and norepinephrine from the adrenal medulla?
   a) Parasympathetic activation b) Sympathetic activation
   c) ACTH from the pituitary d) Increased blood glucose

74. From which part of the brain does the pineal gland develop?
    a) Telencephalon b) Mesencephalon
    c) Diencephalon d) Metencephalon
75. What type of cells differentiate in the developing pineal gland?
    a) Neurons and astrocytes
    b) Pinealocytes and glial cells
    c) Ependymal cells and oligodendrocytes
    d) Microglia and neurons
76. What layer of connective tissue surrounds the developing pineal gland?
    a) Dura mater b) Arachnoid mater
    c) Pia mater d) Gray matter
77. Which hormone is secreted by the pineal gland?
    a) Serotonin b) Dopamine
    c) Cortisol d) Melatonin
78. How does the pineal gland influence the onset of the breeding season in domestic animals?
    a) By increasing cortisol secretion b) Through the release of melatonin
    c) By inhibiting pituitary function d) By decreasing body temperature
79. In what type of breeders does increased exposure to daylight decrease melatonin synthesis?
    a) Short day breeders b) Long day breeders
    c) Continuous day breeders d) Random day breeders
80. Where is melatonin released after being synthesized by pinealocytes?
    a) Into the cerebrospinal fluid b) Directly into the synaptic cleft
    c) Into the lymphatic system d) Into the bile ducts
81. What triggers the increased secretion of melatonin in animals?
    a) Increased daylight exposure b) Increased temperature
    c) Darkness d) Fasting
82. Which structure provides blood supply to the pineal gland?
    a) Pia mater b) Arachnoid mater
    c) Dura mater d) Ventricles
83. The pineal gland's secretion of melatonin is primarily controlled by:
    a) Blood glucose levels
    b) The duration of exposure to light and darkness
    c) Body temperature
    d) Oxygen levels
84. The processes developed by pinealocytes release melatonin into which of the following?
    a) Synaptic clefts b) Lymphatic vessels
    c) Capillaries or cerebrospinal fluid d) Gastrointestinal tract

85. Which of the following best describes the role of melatonin in the pineal gland's function?
   a) It enhances cognitive function
   b) It regulates circadian rhythms and seasonal reproductive cycles
   c) It increases metabolic rate
   d) It stimulates muscle growth
86. Increased exposure to daylight activates sensory neurons in which part of the body?
   a) Retina
   b) Pineal gland
   c) Hypothalamus
   d) Pituitary gland
87. Which hormone is primarily responsible for triggering the release of gonadotrophic hormones in response to melatonin?
   a) Adrenocorticotropic hormone (ACTH)
   b) Thyroid-stimulating hormone (TSH)
   c) Gonadotrophin-releasing hormone (GnRH)
   d) Growth hormone
88. Which of the following statements is true regarding the pineal gland's role in short day breeders?
   a) Melatonin synthesis is suppressed by prolonged daylight
   b) The pineal gland secretes high levels of serotonin
   c) Melatonin synthesis increases with prolonged daylight
   d) The pineal gland has no role in short day breeders
89. The adenohypophysis develops from which of the following?
   a) Neuroectoderm
   b) Oral ectoderm
   c) Mesoderm
   d) Endoderm
90. What is the primordial structure from which the adenohypophysis develops?
   a) Infundibulum
   b) Rathke's pouch
   c) Adenohypophyseal cleft
   d) Pars tuberalis
91. The neurohypophysis develops from which part of the diencephalon?
   a) Roof of the diencephalon
   b) Floor of the diencephalon
   c) Lateral wall of the diencephalon
   d) Caudal end of the diencephalon
92. Which part of the adenohypophysis surrounds the stalk of the infundibulum?
   a) Pars distalis
   b) Pars intermedia
   c) Pars nervosa
   d) Pars tuberalis
93. Which cells in the pars distalis produce growth hormone and prolactin?
   a) Chromophobes
   b) Basophils
   c) Acidophils
   d) Pituicytes
94. Basophils in the pars distalis are responsible for secreting which of the following hormones?
   a) Oxytocin and ADH
   b) ACTH and TSH
   c) Growth hormone and prolactin
   d) Melanocyte-stimulating hormone

95. What is the primary role of chromophobes in the pars distalis?
   a) They are a source of pituicytes
   b) They produce neurohormones
   c) They are either stem cells or non-secreting stages of acidophils or basophils
   d) They secrete melanocyte-stimulating hormone

96. In ruminants, the hypophyseal cleft is:
   a) Obliterated
   b) Persistent
   c) Absent
   d) Fused with the pars distalis

97. In which species is the hypophyseal cleft obliterated?
   a) Carnivores
   b) Pigs
   c) Horses
   d) Ruminants

98. What are pituicytes?
   a) Modified astrocytes in the pars nervosa
   b) Hormone-secreting cells in the pars distalis
   c) Stem cells in the pars tuberalis
   d) Neurons in the infundibulum

99. Which of the following best describes Rathke's pouch?
   a) A midline evagination of neural ectoderm
   b) A dorsal diverticulum from the floor of the diencephalon
   c) A midline evagination of oral ectoderm
   d) A ventral diverticulum from the roof of the diencephalon

100. Which structure differentiates into the pars nervosa?
   a) Rathke's pouch
   b) Adenohypophyseal cleft
   c) Infundibulum
   d) Adenohypophyseal vesicle

101. What is the relationship between the pars intermedia and the pars nervosa in horses, pigs, and carnivores?
   a) The pars intermedia encloses the infundibulum and contacts the surface of the pars nervosa
   b) The pars nervosa surrounds the pars intermedia
   c) The pars intermedia is separate from the pars nervosa
   d) The pars intermedia is fused with the pars distalis

102. Which of the following structures is NOT a component of the neurohypophysis?
   a) Pars nervosa
   b) Infundibulum
   c) Pars intermedia
   d) Hypophyseal stalk

103. Where are the neurosecretions from the supraoptic and paraventricular nuclei stored?
   a) In the pars distalis
   b) In the pars intermedia
   c) In the pars nervosa
   d) In the infundibulum

104. The adenohypophyseal cleft is formed as a result of:
   a) Proliferation of cells in the rostral wall of the adenohypophyseal vesicle
   b) Fusion of the pars distalis with the neural lobe
   c) Obliteration of Rathke's pouch
   d) Migration of neuroepithelial cells

Answer Key

1	a	2	c	3	b	4	b	5	c	6	b	7	b
8	b	9	c	10	c	11	b	12	c	13	d	14	b
15	b	16	a	17	b	18	a	19	c	20	d	21	b
22	c	23	b	24	c	25	c	26	b	27	d	28	b
29	b	30	c	31	c	32	c	33	c	34	b	35	b
36	c	37	b	38	c	39	c	40	b	41	b	42	c
43	c	44	b	45	c	46	c	47	b	48	b	49	a
50	b	51	c	52	b	53	b	54	d	55	b	56	b
57	b	58	c	59	c	60	b	61	b	62	c	63	b
64	b	65	c	66	c	67	b	68	b	69	a	70	c
71	d	72	c	73	b	74	c	75	b	76	c	77	d
78	b	79	a	80	a	81	c	82	a	83	b	84	c
85	b	86	a	87	c	88	a	89	b	90	b	91	b
92	d	93	c	94	b	95	c	96	b	97	c	98	a
99	c	100	c	101	a	102	c	103	c	104	a		

24

Development of Eye and Ear

Rakesh Kumar Barhaiya[1] *and Babita Das*[2]

[1]*Department of Veterinary Anatomy, C.O.V.S.C. & A.H., Jabalpur*

[2]*Department of Veterinary Surgery, C.O.V.S.C. & A.H., Jabalpur*

Introduction

Development of eye

The eyeball is a complex structure having tunics i.e. fibrous tunic (sclera, cornea), vascular tunic (iris, ciliary body, choroid)and nervous tunic (retin a)and its adnexa i.e. eyelids, lacrimal apparatus, extraocular muscles, conjunctiva and other soft tissue are very important structure for proper functioning of eye. The embryonic tissue which contributes for development of eye and its adnexa are:

1. **Surface ectoderm of the head**: Lens, corneal epithelium, eyelids, Lacrimal gland and conjunctival epithelium
2. **Neural ectoderm of the forebrain:** Retina, Posterior epithelium of iris and ciliary body, optic nerve
3. **Mesoderm:** Cornea stroma, Descemet's membrane, Choroid, Sclera, extra-ocular muscles

Development of eye begins simultaneously with the development of brain by the process of neurulation. Neural tube is lined by neuroectoderm and the exterior of embryo lined by surface ectoderm. Neural crest cells, population of specialized mesenchymal cells develop from the lateral border of the neural fold and do not participate in the formation of neural tube. These neural crest cells migrate under the surface ectoderm peripherally and populating the region around the optic vesicle and form the future all connective tissue of structure of eye.

Formation of optic vesicle and optic cup which develop the retina

The optic sulci are visible as paired evaginations of the forebrain neural ectoderm on day 13 of gestation in the dog. The outpouching on either side of optic field of diencephalon (caudal part of prosencephalon) called optic vesicle which attached to the diencephalon by optic stalk. In dog, it appears at the gestation age of day 15. Each optic vesicle grows laterally until it comes into contact with the surface ectoderm. The surface ectoderm become thickened to form the lens placode near the optic vesicle. This lens placode invaginates into the optic vesicles and form lens vesicle, which later on loses it contact with the surface ectoderm. Simultaneously, the optic vesicle invaginates to form double layered optic cups. The neuroepithelial cells of inner layer of the optic cups proliferate and differentiate into rods, cones, bipolar and ganglion cells and glial cells of neural part of the retina and cells of the outer layer become pigmented and form pigmented epithelium of retina)Optic fissure is an area which develops with the progression of optic cup formation from superior to inferiorly where side wall of optic cup meets with the optic stalk. Neural crest cells (mesenchymal cells) fill the surrounding of optic cup and give rise to hyaloid artery in the optic fissure and entered into the optic cup through optic stalk for developing lens. Later on, this optic (foetal) fissure closed through fusion with the optic cup and if persist may result in defect in the iris (colobomas), choroid or optic nerve.

Lens placode and lens vesicle that develop the lens

With the development of optic cup, the lens placode (from surface ectoderm) invaginates into the rim of optic vesicle and forms lens vesicle. Subsequently, the lens vesicle loses its contact with the surface ectoderm (day 25 of gestation in the dog) and surrounded by mesenchymal tissue and becomes positioned at the opening of optic cup. The lens vesicle is lined by a monolayer of cuboidal cells surrounded by a basal lamina)

Development of the Cornea, Anterior Chamber, Sclera and Choroid

The foetal cornea has complex structure, histologically formed by

1. Anterior epithelium: developed from surface ectoderm
2. Primary stroma: developed from mesenchymal cells (derived from neural crest) present surroundings to the optic cup.
3. Corneal endothelium: developed from mesenchymal cells

The mesenchymal cells derived from neural crest present in the region between the lens and surface ectoderm, arranged into two layers and the resultant cavity become anterior chamber. The outer layer becomes substantia propria and mesothelium of cornea and sclera also develop from it. The choroid and sclera are relatively differentiated at birth, but the tapetum in dogs and cats continues to develop and mature during the first 4 months postnatally. The inner layer of these mesenchymal cells differentiated into the highly vascularized pigmented layer of choroid The posterior chamber of the eye arises from a space that forms in the mesenchyme posterior to the developing iris and anterior to the developing lens. When the pupillary membrane disappears, anterior and posterior chambers of the eye can communicate with each other through the pupil opening.

Vitreous body

Except in pigs, a refractive tapetum lucidum is formed in the choroid layer of herbivores and carnivores. Some of the loose mesenchymal tissue which surrounds the optic cup migrates to the position between the retina and lens to form vitreous body which receives blood supply from branches of hyaloid artery. Later this artery atrophies and the space occupied by the artery becomes hyaloid canal.

Development of Iris, Ciliary body and Irido-corneal angle

The iris stroma develops from the anterior segment mesenchymal tissue (neural crest cell origin), and the iris pigmented and nonpigmented epithelia originate from the neural ectoderm of the optic cup. The smooth muscles of the pupillary sphincter and dilator muscles ultimately differentiate from these epithelial layers, and they represent the only mammalian muscles of neural ectodermal origin. In avian species, however, the skeletal muscle cells in the iris are of neural crest origin, with a possible small contribution of mesoderm to the ventral portion. The ciliary body epithelium develops from the neuroectoderm of the anterior optic cup, and the underlying mesenchyme differentiates into the ciliary muscles.

Development of eyelid and extraocular muscles

The eyelids develop from surface ectoderm, which gives rise to the epidermis, cilia, and conjunctival epithelium. Neural crest mesenchyme gives rise to deeper structures, including the dermis and tarsus. The eyelid muscles (i.e., orbicularis and levator) are derived from craniofacial condensations of mesoderm called somitomeres. The upper eyelid develops from the frontonasal process; the lower eyelid develops from the maxillary process. The lid folds grow together and elongate to cover the developing eye. The upper and lower lids fuse on day 32 of gestation in the dog. Separation occurs 2 weeks postnatally. The extraocular muscles arise from mesoderm in somitomeres (i.e., preoptic mesodermal condensations). The axons of the ganglion cells infiltrate the optic stalk and form optic nerve.

Development of Ear

The internal ear develops from the bilateral thickenings of the surface ectoderm (otic placode) at the level of myelencephalon. Under the influence of growth factor, the otic placodes invaginate to form the otic pits, which make contact with the wall of the myelencephalon. Later on, otic vesicle develops and separated it from the surface ectoderm. This otic vesicle filled with endolymph. A finger-like evagination of the otic vesicle gives rise to the endolymphatic duct and its terminal structure called endolymphatic sa c) The otic vesicle differentiated into utricle and saccule dorsally and ventrally respectively. Semicircular duct develops from utricle. Cochlear duct develops from the saccule. The connection between the saccule and the cochlea becomes constricted and forms the narrow ductus reuniens. The cartilaginous labyrinth develops by surrounded mesenchymal tissue.

The tympanic cavity and the Eustachian tube develops from an expansion of the first pharyngeal pouch, between the first and second pharyngeal arches and therefore it is lined by epithelium of endoderm in origin. The malleus and incus develop from neural-crest-derived mesenchyme of the first pharyngeal arch, whereas the stapes originates from the second pharyngeal arch mesenchyme. The structure of tympanic membrane originated from all three-germ layer. The auricles are formed from mesenchymal tissue of the first and second pharyngeal arches that surround the first pharyngeal cleft.

Multiple Choice Questions

1. Development of eye start from which part of the neural tube
   - a) Telencephalon
   - b) Diencephalon
   - c) Mesencephalon
   - d) Rhombencephalon
2. The neural plate (neuroectoderm) originated from...............
   - a) Epiblast cells anterior to primitive node
   - b) Epiblast cells posterior to primitive node
   - c) Hypoblast cells
   - d) None

3. The neural tube is line by
   a) Neuroectoderm b) Surface ectoderm
   c) Mesoderm d) Endoderm
4. Development of eye begins with formation of ....
   a) Optic sulci b) Optic vesicle
   c) Otic placode d) Lens placode
5. The embryonic tissue which contributes to the formation of eye.........
   a) Neuroectoderm
   b) Surface ectoderm
   c) Neural crest derived mesenchymal cell
   d) All of the above
6. The optic vesicle are visible as paired evaginations of the forebrain neural ectoderm, on day............... of gestation in dog
   a) 11 b) 12
   c) 13 d) 14
7. The outpouching on either side of optic field of diencephalon (caudal part of prosencephalon) called.........
   a) Otic placode b) Optic vesicle
   c) Optic stalk d) Lens placode
8. Lens placode develops from the......
   a) Surface ectoderm near optic vesicle b) Neuroectoderm
   c) Neural crest cells d) Optic sulci
9. The optic vesicle invaginates to form double layered structure called ....
   a) Lens placode b) Optic cup
   c) Optic stalk d) Lens
10. The neuroepithelial cells of inner layer of the optic cups proliferate and differentiate into..............
    a) Retina b) Lens
    c) Choroid d) Iris
11. The neuroepithelial cells of outer layer of the optic cups proliferate and differentiate into..............
    a) Retina b) Ciliary body
    c) Retinal pigmented epithelium d) Choroid
12. The hyaloid artery develops at the age of....................gestation in dog
    a) 25 b) 30
    c) 35 d) 40
13. Mesenchymal tissue of eye develops from the
    a) Surface ectoderm b) Neuroectoderm
    c) Neural crest cells d) All

14. The hyaloid artery develops from the
   a) Optic cup
   b) Optic stalk
   c) Optic fissure
   d) Mesenchymal tissue
15. ....is an area where optic cup and optic stalk meets inferiorly with progression of invagination of lens placode/optic vesicle
   a) Coloboma
   b) Otic fissure
   c) Optic fissure
   d) None of the above
16. The hyaloid artery courses from ....
   a) Lens placode to the optic cup
   b) Optic stalk to the lens placode (developing lens)
   c) Both
   d) None of the above
17. Failure in closure of optic fissure may cause
   a) Defect in retina
   b) Defects in lens
   c) Defects in iris (coloboma), optic nerve and choroid
   d) All
18. Lens development begins with the thickening of the lens placode at the age of ....day of gestation in dog
   a) 17
   b) 20
   c) 23
   d) 26
19. The lens placode invaginates into the rim of optic vesicle and forms a hollow sphere called ....
   a) Vitreous
   b) Lens vesicle
   c) Lens node
   d) Lens epithelium
20. The lens vesicle loses its contact with the surface ectoderm at the age of ....day of gestation in dog
   a) 20
   b) 25
   c) 30
   d) 45
21. The lens vesicle is lined by...................
   a) Monolayer of cuboidal cells with basal lamina
   b) Monolayer of cuboidal cells without basal lamina
   c) Bilayer of cuboidal cells
   d) Monolayer of columnar cells
22. Lens capsule develops from
   a) Primitive retina
   b) Basal lamina of anterior cuboidal cells
   c) Basal lamina of retinal pigmented epithelium
   d) None of the above

23. Aplasia of lens may result from
    a) Failure of lens induction
    b) Failure of involution of lens vesicle
    c) Failure of separation of lens vesicle from the surface ectoderm
    d) All of the above
24. The embryonic lens fibres have features.................
    a) The embryonic lens fibres are the embryonic lens nucleus
    b) The primitive retina promotes primary lens formation near anterior epithelium
    c) In adult, no sutures in the embryonic nucleus
    d) All of the above
25. In adult, the secondary lens fibres develop from..............
    a) Posteriors lens capsule b) Anterior lens capsule
    c) Anterior epithelium d) None of the above
26. The anterior epithelium of lens have features...................
    a) The anterior epithelium is simple cuboidal type
    b) It has mitotic activity throughout the life
    c) It forms lens cells (fibres) of lens cortex
    d) All of the above
27. The primary lens fibres develop from........
    a) Anterior cuboidal epithelium of developing lens
    b) Elongation of epithelial cells from the posterior pole of lens vesicle
    c) Both a and b
    d) None of the above
28. The secondary lens fibres develop from ....
    a) Elongation of anterior lens epithelium
    b) Elongation of posterior lens capsule
    c) Elongation of anterior lens capsule
    d) None of the above
29. The factors which affect the development of lens ....
    a) Fibroblast like growth factor from retina
    b) Blood supply from vessels of stroma of iris (pupillary membrane) for the anterior surface
    c) Blood supply from hyaloid artery for the posterior surface
    d) All of the above
30. The developing cornea has following layer.........
    a) Anterior epithelium b) Corneal stroma
    c) Corneal endothelium d) All of the above

31. The anterior epithelium of cornea develops from ....
    a) Surface ectoderm overlying the optic cup
    b) Mesenchymal neural crest cells surrounding the optic cup
    c) Both a and b
    d) None of the above

32. The primary stroma of cornea develops from
    a) Posterior pigmented epithelium of iris b) Mesenchymal neural crest cells
    c) Surface ectoderm d) All of the above

33. The anterior chamber is the space between ....
    a) Between corneal endothelium to the anterior surface of iris
    b) Between posterior surface of iris and anterior surface of lens
    c) Between the posterior surface of lens and retina
    d) None of the above

34. The anterior chamber develops from the ....
    a) It arises from a space that forms in the mesenchyme posterior to the developing iris and anterior to the developing lens
    b) It arises from a space within the mesenchymal tissue between the developing cornea and the lens
    c) It arises from a space within the mesenchymal tissue between the developing lens and retina
    d) Both a and b

35. Corneal endothelium develops from
    a) Surface ectoderm b) Mesenchymal neural crest cells
    c) Neuroectoderm d) None of the above

36. Posterior epithelium of iris and ciliary body develops from
    a) Neuroectoderm of optic cup b) Mesoderm
    c) Surface ectoderm d) All of the above

37. Pigmented and non-pigmented epithelium of iris and ciliary body develops from ....
    a) Anterior aspect of optic cup b) Posterior aspect of optic cup
    c) Both a and b d) None of the above

38. The iris stroma develops from
    a) Mesenchymal cell b) Neuroectoderm
    c) Surface ectoderm d) All of the above

39. The smooth muscles of the pupillary sphincter and dilator muscles have .... origine
    a) Neuroectoderm b) Mesoderm
    c) Surface ectoderm d) Endoderm

40. Suspensory ligament of the lens develops from
    a) Mesenchymal cell between the ciliary process and lens
    b) Ectodermal cells
    c) Mesodermal cells
    d) Endodermal cells
41. The eyelids develop from ...
    a) Surface ectoderm
    b) Mesenchymal neural crest cells
    c) Both a and b
    d) None of the above
42. The separation of eyelids occurs at ....in canines
    a) About 8-10 days pre-natally
    b) About 8-10 days post-natally
    c) About 12-14 days pre-natally
    d) About 12-14 days post-natally
43. The extra-ocular muscles develop from
    a) Mesenchymal cells
    b) Mesoderm in somitomeres
    c) Endoderm
    d) Ectoderm
44. The separation of eyelids occurs at ....in humans
    a) About 7 months of gestation
    b) About 8 months of gestation
    c) About 7 days post-natally
    d) About 7 days pre-natally
45. Optic axon (nerve) develops from which cells of the retina......
    a) Ganglion cell
    b) Amacrine cells
    c) Mullers cells
    d) Glial cells
46. The tapetum usually differentiated at birth in domestic animals but in dog and cats it mature at........
    a) Mature fully at 10 days pre-natally
    b) Mature fully at 10 days post -natally
    c) Mature during the first 4 months postnatally
    d) Mature during the first 1 months postnatally
47. Congenital anomalies in which all or part of the margin of eyelid is turned inwards
    a) Ectropion
    b) Entropion
    c) Coloboma
    d) Cyclopia
48. Cyclopia is a congenital anomaly characterized by ...
    a) Fused right and left globes
    b) Single median globe
    c) Abnormal ocular size
    d) Failure of optic fissure closure
49. After regression of hyaloid artery, the remnants of hyaloid vasculature and some glial tissue may emanate from the optic disc and it can be viewed ophthalmoscopically called...
    a) Bergmeiter's papilla
    b) Vaculosa lentis
    c) Hyaloid canal
    d) None of the above
50. A fold of mesenchyme covered by conjunctiva at the medial angle of eye forms...
    a) Lacrimal gland
    b) Naso-lacrimal duct
    c) Third eyelid
    d) Ciliary processes

51. Coloboma is a congenital disorder due to abnormal closure of optic (choroid) fissure, characterized by

a) Aniridia
b) Dyscoria
c) Choroidal hypoplasia
d) All of the above

52. Microphakia is characterized by

a) Small lens
b) Small Optic disc
c) Narrow pupillary opening
d) Small eye

53. The schelmm's canal is responsible for

a) Drainage of vitreous humour
b) Drainage of aqueous humour
c) Maintaining intraocular pressure
d) Both c and d

54. Lacrimal glands from .....

a) Mesoderm
b) Endoderm
c) Surface ectoderm
d) Mesenchymal cells

55. The clinical lens anomaly in which a small area of fibrosis seen on the posterior lens capsule called ......

a) Mitten-dorf's dot
b) Bergmeiter's papilla
c) Vaculosa lentis
d) None of the above

56. What are the congenital anomalies of the eye......

a) Abnormal formation of primary and secondary lens fibres leads to cataract
b) Malformation of the irido-corneal angle leads to glaucoma
c) Persistent hyperplastic primary vitreous
d) All of the above

57. The inner ear develops from the

a) Bilateral ectodermal thickenings at the level of rhombencephalon
b) Bilateral ectodermal thickenings at the level of Mesencephalon
c) Bilateral ectodermal thickenings at the level of telencephalon
d) First pharyngeal pouch

58. The external ear consists of ......

a) Auricle
b) External auditory meatus
c) External layer of tympanic membrane
d) All of the above

59. Bilateral ectodermal thickenings at the level of rhombencephalon called

a) Lens placode
b) Otic placode
c) Otic swelling
d) None of the above

60. After loosing connection with the ectoderm otic placode became ....

a) Otic vesicle filled with endolymph
b) Otic vesicle filled with perilymph
c) Utricle
d) Saccule

61. Otic vesicle (otocyst) to be differentiated first into .... distinct region
   a) Dorsally saccule and ventrally utricle
   b) Dorsally utricle and ventrally saccule
   c) Semicircular duct and cochlear duct
   d) None of the above

62. A finger-like evagination of the dorsomedial region of the otic vesicle gives rise to..
   a) Endolymphatic duct b) Anterior semicircular duct
   c) Posterior semicircular duct d) None of the above

63. The cochlear diverticulum evaginates from the ....
   a) Dorsal part of saccule b) Ventral part of saccule
   c) Dorsal part of utricle d) Ventral part of utricle

64. The anterior and posterior semicircular duct develops from the........
   a) Two disc like diverticulum from the saccule
   b) Two disc like diverticulum from the utricle
   c) Cochleovestibular duct
   d) None of the above

65. The central part of the horizontal and vertical disc became ....
   a) Over grown to form later semicircular duct
   b) Became undergrown for apoptosis
   c) Nothing will happen to the central part of these disc
   d) None of the above

66. All semicircular ducts are at the .... degree angle to each other
   a) 90 b) 45
   c) 180 d) 270

67. Crista ampularis is the specialized sensory structure found in ....
   a) At the tip of cochlear duct
   b) Enlarge part of the semicircular duct at its junction with the utricle
   c) At the mid part of each semicircular duct
   d) All of the above

68. The sensory organs for the body balance
   a) Macula utricle b) Macula saccule
   c) Crista ampularis d) All of the above

69. The connection between the saccule and the cochlea becomes constricted and forms the ....
   a) Ductus reunion b) Endolymphatic duct
   c) Endolymphatic sac d) All of the above

70. The cartilaginous labyrinth is formed by ....
   a) Neuroectoderm b) Mesenchymal cells
   c) Endoderm d) Surface ectoderm

71. The space between embryonic vestibular/cochlear membranous and cartilage called)..
   a) Endolymphatic space
   b) Perilymphatic space
   c) Scala tympani
   d) Scala vestibuli
72. The external auditory meatus derives from ....
   a) An outward expansion of the first pharyngeal cleft
   b) An inward expansion of the first pharyngeal cleft
   c) An outward expansion of the first pharyngeal pouch
   d) An inward expansion of the first pharyngeal pouch
73. At the beginning of development of external auditory meatus, it is........
   a) Hollow tube and need of canalization
   b) Solid tube and became hollow tube through canalization
   c) Both a and b
   d) Neither a or b
74. Tympanic membrane originates from
   a) Ectoderm
   b) Mesoderm
   c) Endoderm
   d) All of the above
75. The auricle develops from ......
   a) Mesenchymal tissue of first pharyngeal arch
   b) Mesenchymal tissue of second pharyngeal arch
   c) Both a and b
   d) None of the above
76. The middle ear cavity (tympanic cavity) and eustachian tube develops from
   a) An expansion of first pharyngeal pouch between the first and second pharyngeal arch
   b) An expansion of second pharyngeal pouch between the second and third pharyngeal arch
   c) An expansion of third pharyngeal pouch between the third and fourth pharyngeal arch
   d) All of the above
77. The middle ear cavity and eustachian tube are lined by ....
   a) Ectoderm derived epithelium
   b) Mesoderm derived epithelium
   c) Endoderm derived epithelium
   d) All of the above
78. In equine, ventral diverticulum of eustachian tube called.....
   a) Crop
   b) Guttural pouch
   c) Ear drum
   d) None of the above
79. The malleus and incus develop from the...
   a) Mesenchymal neural crest cells of first pharyngeal pouch
   b) Mesenchymal neural crest cells of second pharyngeal pouch
   c) Mesenchymal neural crest cells of third pharyngeal pouch
   d) All of the above

80. The stapes (ear ossicle) develops from the...
 a) Mesenchymal neural crest cells of first pharyngeal pouch
 b) Mesenchymal neural crest cells of second pharyngeal pouch
 c) Mesenchymal neural crest cells of third pharyngeal pouch
 d) All of the above

Answer Key

1	b	2	a	3	a	4	a	5	d	6	c	7	b
8	a	9	b	10	a	11	c	12	a	13	c	14	d
15	c	16	b	17	c	18	a	19	b	20	b	21	a
22	b	23	d	24	d	25	c	26	d	27	b	28	a
29	d	30	d	31	a	32	b	33	a	34	b	35	b
36	a	37	a	38	a	39	a	40	a	41	c	42	b
43	b	44	a	45	a	46	c	47	b	48	b	49	a
50	c	51	d	52	a	53	d	54	c	55	a	56	d
57	a	58	d	59	b	60	a	61	b	62	a	63	b
64	b	65	b	66	a	67	b	68	d	69	a	70	b
71	b	72	c	73	b	74	d	75	c	76	a	77	c
78	b	79	a	80	b								

25

Age Determination of Embryo and Foetus

Jasvinder Singh Sasan, Kamal Sarma and Shalini Suri

Division of Veterinary Anatomy, Faculty of Veterinary Sciences and Animal Husbandry, Sher-e-Kashmir University of Agricultural Sciences and Technology of Jammu, Jammu and Kashmir

After fertilization and zygote formation, in utero development can be divided into two stages, i.e. embryonic and foetal. Embryo period refers to the time between fertilization and the development of organ primordia. During the embryonic period, fast development occurs, and primordia of most organs are established. During the foetal stage, which lasts from the end of the embryonic period until parturition, the body's systems begin to develop and function.

Multiple Choice Questions

1. At the end of gastrulation, developing embryo is:
   - a) Elongated　　b) Pear shaped
   - c) Oval　　d) Cylindrical
2. The embryonic period is defined as the interval from:
   - a) Fertilization to birth
   - b) Fertilization to development of organ primordia
   - c) Development of organ primordia to birth
   - d) None of the above
3. Embryonic period in sheep is approximately:
   - a) 30 days　　b) 50 days
   - c) 56 days　　d) 60 days
4. The foetal period is defined as the interval from:
   - a) Fertilization to birth
   - b) Fertilization to development of organ primordia
   - c) Development of organ primordia to birth
   - d) None of the above
5. Embryonic period in dog is approximately:
   - a) 30 days　　b) 50 days
   - c) 56 days　　d) 60 days

6. Embryonic period in cattle is approximately:
   a) 30 days b) 50 days
   c) 56 days d) 60 days
7. Which is incorrect about embryonic period of cattle:
   a) Primordia of most organs are established
   b) Approximately of 56 days
   c) Extends up to parturition
   d) All are correct
8. Embryonic period in horses is approximately:
   a) 30 days b) 50 days
   c) 56 days d) 60 days
9. Embryonic period in pig is approximately:
   a) 30 days b) 50 days
   c) 56 days d) 60 days
10. Embryonic period in humans is approximately:
   a) 30 days b) 50 days
   c) 56 days d) 60 days
11. Growth and initiation of physiological functioning of body systems is characteristic feature of:
   a) Embryonic period b) Foetal period
   c) Both a & b d) None of the above
12. Average gestation length of cattle is:
   a) 278 days b) 335 days
   c) 310 days d) 150 days
13. Average gestation length of buffalo is:
   a) 278 days b) 335 days
   c) 310 days d) 150 days
14. Average gestation length of horse is:
   a) 278 days b) 335 days
   c) 310 days d) 150 days
15. Average gestation length of goat is:
   a) 278 days b) 335 days
   c) 310 days d) 150 days
16. Average gestation length of pig is:
   a) 114 days b) 335 days
   c) 310 days d) 150 days
17. Average gestation length of sheep is:
   a) 148 days b) 335 days
   c) 310 days d) 278 days

18. In cattle, 1st pair of somite appears at what stage of gestation:
 a) 10th day of gestation b) 20th day of gestation
 c) 30th day of gestation d) 40th day of gestation
19. In cattle, three brain vesicles appears at what stage of gestation:
 a) 10th day of gestation b) 24th day of gestation
 c) 30th day of gestation d) 44th day of gestation
20. In sheep, 1st pair of somite appears at what stage of gestation:
 a) 10th day of gestation b) 15th day of gestation
 c) 20th day of gestation d) 24th day of gestation
21. In pig, primitive streak appears at what stage of gestation:
 a) 12th day of gestation b) 20th day of gestation
 c) 24th day of gestation d) 40th day of gestation
22. In dog, 1st pair of somite appears at what stage of gestation:
 a) 10th day of gestation b) 16th day of gestation
 c) 20th day of gestation d) 24th day of gestation
23. In cattle, primitive streak appears at what stage of gestation:
 a) 10th day of gestation b) 14th day of gestation
 c) 20th day of gestation d) 24th day of gestation
24. In cattle, initiation of placentation appears at what stage of gestation:
 a) 10th day of gestation b) 14th day of gestation
 c) 19th day of gestation d) 24th day of gestation
25. In sheep, initiation of placentation appears at what stage of gestation:
 a) 10th day of gestation b) 15th day of gestation
 c) 30th day of gestation d) 24th day of gestation

Answer Key

1	b	2	b	3	a	4	c	5	a	6	c	7	c
8	c	9	a	10	c	11	b	12	a	13	c	14	b
15	d	16	a	17	a	18	b	19	b	20	b	21	a
22	b	23	b	24	c	25	b						

26

Teratology

Ersavadla Rajaraviteja[1] and Suvaneeth P.[2]

[1]Department of Veterinary Anatomy, Faculty of Veterinary and Animal Sciences Institute of Agricultural Sciences, Rajiv Gandhi South Campus, Banaras Hindu University, Barkachha, Mirzapur-231001

[2]Department of Veterinary Pathology, Faculty of Veterinary and Animal Sciences, Institute of Agricultural Sciences, Rajiv Gandhi South Campus, Banaras Hindu University, Barkachha, Mirzapur-231001

Introduction

Teratology is the branch of veterinary embryology that studies congenital malformations, often referred to as birth defects, which arise during embryonic or fetal development. Understanding teratology is crucial for veterinarians and researchers because these defects can lead to substantial animal morbidity, mortality, and economic losses in the agricultural and livestock industries. In addition, teratological research can offer insights into human congenital disorders, given the similarities between mammalian developmental processes.

Definition and Scope of Teratology

The term "teratology" derives from the Greek word *teras*, meaning "monster" or "marvel," reflecting the historical observation of grossly abnormal fetuses or neonates. Teratology focuses on the etiology (causes), pathogenesis (development), and morphological consequences of developmental disorders. These abnormalities can manifest as structural, functional, or biochemical anomalies, and they can affect a wide range of systems, including the cardiovascular, skeletal, nervous, and reproductive systems.

In veterinary medicine, the study of teratogens—agents that cause developmental malformations—is critical. Teratogens include drugs, environmental chemicals, infections, radiation, and nutritional deficiencies, among others. These agents can disrupt normal embryonic or fetal development, leading to a variety of abnormalities.

Causes of Teratogenesis

Teratogenic agents can be broadly classified into several categories:

1. Genetic Factors

Genetic mutations, chromosomal abnormalities, and hereditary disorders can predispose animals to developmental defects. Genetic teratogenesis can occur due to spontaneous mutations in the DNA sequence or inheritance of defective genes from one or both parents. Chromosomal anomalies, such as duplications, deletions, or translocations of genetic material, can also cause significant malformations. For instance, certain skeletal abnormalities and metabolic disorders in animals are linked to specific genetic mutations.

2. Infectious Agents

Certain viral, bacterial, and protozoal infections during pregnancy can lead to teratogenic outcomes. Viruses such as bovine viral diarrhea virus (BVDV), feline panleukopenia virus, and porcine parvovirus are known to cross the placenta and infect the developing embryo or fetus. These infections can cause abortion, mummification of the fetus, or severe malformations such as cerebellar hypoplasia, hydrocephalus, and skeletal deformities.

Protozoal infections like Toxoplasma gondii in small ruminants can also cause congenital malformations or fetal death, depending on the stage of gestation when infection occurs. These infectious agents often disrupt cell proliferation, differentiation, and tissue patterning, leading to developmental arrest or abnormal organogenesis.

3. Chemical and Environmental Teratogens

Numerous chemicals and environmental factors are known to interfere with embryonic and fetal development. These agents include industrial pollutants, pesticides, heavy metals, and veterinary drugs. For example, ingestion of certain toxic plants, such as *Veratrum californicum* by pregnant livestock, can result in congenital deformities, particularly cyclopia (one-eyed fetus) in sheep. Similarly, exposure to certain pesticides or herbicides during pregnancy can lead to defects in the cardiovascular, nervous, and skeletal systems of animals.

Heavy metals like lead, mercury, and cadmium are also potent teratogens that can affect neural tube development, limb formation, and other critical developmental processes. Radiation exposure, either through diagnostic imaging or environmental sources, can disrupt cell division and DNA synthesis, resulting in malformations or pregnancy loss.

4. Nutritional Deficiencies

Nutritional imbalances or deficiencies during pregnancy are a well-known cause of congenital malformations in animals. One of the most extensively studied examples is vitamin A deficiency in cattle and pigs, which leads to defects in organ development, particularly the eye, heart, and nervous system. Vitamin A is essential for normal cell differentiation and tissue patterning during embryogenesis.

Folate deficiency is another significant contributor to neural tube defects in many species, including livestock. Folate is crucial for DNA synthesis and cell division, and its deficiency can result in incomplete closure of the neural tube, leading to conditions such as spina bifida and anencephaly.

5. Physical Factors

Physical factors such as trauma, hyperthermia (elevated maternal body temperature), and uterine crowding can also contribute to teratogenesis. Trauma to the developing fetus, particularly during early gestation, can cause physical deformities or fetal loss. Hyperthermia, often resulting from fever or environmental heat stress, can disrupt normal protein folding and cell division, leading to neural tube defects or limb malformations.

Timing of Teratogen Exposure

The stage of embryonic or fetal development during which exposure to a teratogen occurs is critical in determining the nature and severity of the defect. Embryogenesis can be divided into several key stages, including fertilization, cleavage, gastrulation, organogenesis, and fetal growth. Teratogenic effects are most pronounced during the period of organogenesis, when the basic structures of the organs and tissues are forming. This period, often referred to as the "critical period," is species-specific but generally corresponds to the first third of pregnancy.

- **Pre-implantation phase**: Teratogenic exposure during this phase, typically the first few days after fertilization, may result in the death of the embryo or have no effect at all due to the lack of differentiation.
- **Organogenesis**: This phase is particularly vulnerable to teratogens, as cells are rapidly proliferating and differentiating to form the organs and tissues. Exposure to teratogens during this period can cause a wide range of malformations, depending on which tissues or organ systems are affected)
- **Fetal period**: During the later stages of development, the fetus is generally less sensitive to teratogens, as most organ systems have already formed) However, exposure to certain agents during this period can still result in functional abnormalities, growth retardation, or minor morphological defects.

Common Teratogenic Defects in Veterinary Practice

Several congenital abnormalities frequently observed in veterinary practice include:

1. Limb Malformations

Limb deformities, such as micromelia (short limbs), amelia (absence of limbs), or syndactyly (fusion of digits), can arise due to disruptions in the limb bud during early development. Environmental teratogens like thalidomide or viral infections may interfere with the normal patterning of the limb bud, leading to these defects.

2. Cleft Palate

Cleft palate is a common congenital malformation in animals, particularly in dogs and pigs. It occurs when the two halves of the palate fail to fuse during development, resulting in an opening between the oral and nasal cavities. Genetic factors, nutritional deficiencies, and exposure to certain teratogens during the critical period of palatal fusion contribute to this defect.

3. Neural Tube Defects

Neural tube defects, such as spina bifida and anencephaly, are caused by the incomplete closure of the neural tube during early embryogenesis. These defects can result from genetic mutations, folate deficiency, or exposure to environmental teratogens like heat stress or certain drugs.

4. Cardiac Malformations

Congenital heart defects, such as ventricular septal defects (VSDs) or patent ductus arteriosus (PDa), can arise from disruptions in the early development of the cardiovascular system. Viral infections, nutritional deficiencies, and genetic factors are common causes of these malformations.

Diagnosis and Prevention of Teratogenic Defects

In veterinary practice, diagnosing congenital malformations often involves clinical examination, radiography, ultrasonography, and sometimes genetic testing. Preventative measures include minimizing exposure to known teratogens, ensuring proper maternal nutrition, and vaccinating against infectious agents that can cause teratogenic effects.

For livestock and companion animals, reducing the risk of teratogenesis involves strict management practices, such as avoiding exposure to toxic plants, chemicals, and radiation during pregnancy. Proper vaccination programs and nutritional supplementation, especially with folic acid and vitamin A, can also reduce the incidence of congenital defects.

Conclusion

Teratology, a critical aspect of veterinary embryology, focuses on understanding the causes and consequences of congenital malformations in animals. Teratogens, which range from genetic mutations to infectious agents, chemical toxins, and nutritional deficiencies, disrupt normal embryonic development and result in a variety of structural and functional defects. By understanding the mechanisms of teratogenesis, veterinarians can better diagnose, treat, and prevent congenital disorders, ultimately improving animal health and welfare.

Multiple Choice Questions

1. What is teratology?
   a) Study of plant growth
   b) Study of congenital abnormalities
   c) Study of animal reproduction
   d) Study of viral diseases
2. Which of the following is considered a teratogen?
   a) Antibiotics
   b) Nutritional supplements
   c) Radiation
   d) Water
3. During which stage of embryonic development are embryos most susceptible to teratogens?
   a) Pre-implantation
   b) Organogenesis
   c) Fetal period
   d) Postnatal
4. Which vitamin deficiency is associated with congenital defects like blindness and skeletal malformations in animals?
   a) Vitamin C
   b) VitaminD
   c) Vitamin A
   d) Vitamin E
5. What type of congenital malformation is cyclopia?
   a) Missing limbs
   b) Single eye in the center of the face
   c) Fused digits
   d) Absent tail
6. Thalidomide, a known teratogen, is most associated with which type of birth defect?
   a) Heart defects
   b) Limb malformations
   c) Neural tube defects
   d) Eye defects

7. What is the result of a cleft palate in animals?
   a) Deformation of the limbs
   b) Incomplete fusion of the oral cavity
   c) Absence of tail
   d) Fused digits
8. Which term describes the failure of the neural tube to close completely during development?
   a) Hydrocephalus
   b) Anencephaly
   c) Spina bifida
   d) Holoprosencephaly
9. Which virus is known to cause cerebellar hypoplasia in kittens if the mother is infected during pregnancy?
   a) Canine parvovirus
   b) Feline panleukopenia virus
   c) Bovine viral diarrhea virus
   d) Rabies virus
10. Which congenital abnormality is characterized by an extra number of digits?
   a) Syndactyly
   b) Polydactyly
   c) Micromelia
   d) Amelia
11. Which infectious agent is a known teratogen causing abortion and congenital defects in livestock?
   a) E.col
   b) Toxoplasma gondii
   c) Staphylococcus aureus
   d) Bacillus anthracis
12. Hyperthermia during pregnancy can lead to which type of malformations?
   a) Limb malformations
   b) Neural tube defects
   c) Cardiac malformations
   d) Skin lesions
13. Which plant is known to cause cyclopia in sheep when consumed during pregnancy?
   a) Veratrum californicum
   b) Oleander
   c) Nightshade
   d) Hemlock
14. Teratogens typically affect the fetus most severely during which trimester of pregnancy?
   a) First
   b) Second
   c) Third
   d) Postnatal
15. What is anencephaly?
   a) Malformation of the limbs
   b) Absence of major portions of the brain and skull
   c) Fusion of digits
   d) Development of extra limbs
16. Which of the following is NOT a known cause of congenital malformations?
   a) Genetics
   b) Nutritional deficiency
   c) Aging
   d) Viral infections

17. Folic acid deficiency during pregnancy can lead to which type of defects?
    a) Cleft palate
    b) Limb deformities
    c) Neural tube defects
    d) Cardiac malformations
18. Congenital cardiac defects are most commonly associated with which of the following?
    a) Radiation exposure
    b) Folate deficiency
    c) Viral infections
    d) Genetic mutations
19. What is the most common manifestation of cleft palate in animals?
    a) Difficulty
    b) Difficulty suckling
    c) Legdeformity
    d) Extra digits
20. Which nutrient, if deficient, is most likely to lead to skeletal malformations in developing embryos?
    a) Vitamin C
    b) Vitamin D
    c) Iron
    d) Vitamin B12
21. Which drug is a known teratogen that can cause craniofacial abnormalities in developing animals?
    a) Ivermectin
    b) Griseofulvin
    c) Aspirin
    d) Tetracycline
22. A congenital defect involving the fusion of digits is termed as what?
    a) Polydactyly
    b) Syndactyly
    c) Brachydactyly
    d) Phocomelia
23. Which substance can cause fetal alcohol syndrome in animals?
    a) Ethylene glycol
    b) Ethanol
    c) Caffeine
    d) Nicotine
24. Which environmental condition can lead to developmental malformations in reptiles?
    a) Cold temperatures
    b) UV radiation
    c) Oxygen deficiency
    d) Overheating
25. Spina bifida is a failure of which part of the embryo to close properly?
    a) Neural tube
    b) Limb buds
    c) Cardiovascular system
    d) Gut tube
26. Which of the following is a known effect of lead exposure during pregnancy in animals?
    a) Blindness
    b) Neurological defects
    c) Heart defects
    d) Increased body size
27. Which congenital abnormality is characterized by incomplete development of the cerebellum?
    a) Spina bifida
    b) Hydrocephalus
    c) Cerebellar hypoplasia
    d) Cleft palate

28. Which of the following is a common teratogenic effect of rubella virus in animals?
    a) Cardiac malformations
    b) Neural tube defects
    c) Eye defects
    d) Skeletal malformations
29. Holoprosencephaly is a congenital defect affecting which part of the embryo?
    a) Spinal cord
    b) Brain
    c) Heart
    d) Lungs
30. What is the main teratogenic effect of bovine viral diarrhea virus (BVDV) infection during early pregnancy?
    a) Heart defects
    b) Cerebellar hypoplasia
    c) Abortion
    d) Limb deformities
31. Which nutrient is essential to prevent neural tube defects in embryos?
    a) Vitamin A
    b) Vitamin C
    c) Folic acid
    d) Calcium
32. Which of the following congenital conditions is characterized by an accumulation of fluid in the brain?
    a) Hydrocephalus
    b) Anencephaly
    c) Spina bifida
    d) Holoprosencephaly
33. Which drug, when given to pregnant animals, is known to cause dental and skeletal malformations?
    a) Penicillin
    b) Tetracycline
    c) Aspirin
    d) Amoxicillin
34. The term "amelia" refers to the absence of which of the following?
    a) Skull
    b) Limbs
    c) Tail
    d) Eyes
35. Which teratogenic virus is known to cause microphthalmia (small eyes) in infected animals?
    a) Porcine parvovirus
    b) Rabies virus
    c) Canine distemper virus
    d) Feline leukemia virus
36. Which of the following describes the impact of radiation exposure on embryonic development?
    a) Accelerated growth
    b) Developmental retardation and malformations
    c) Enhanced immunity
    d) Improved cardiovascular function
37. What is the cause of congenital defects in lambs born with cyclopia?
    a) Genetic mutation
    b) Maternal consumption of toxic plants
    c) Viral infection
    d) Vitamin A deficiency

38. A defect in the closure of the abdominal wall leading to herniation of abdominal organs is termed:
   a) Omphalocele b) Cleft palate
   c) Anencephaly d) Polydactyly

39. Which of the following is a teratogenic effect of maternal hyperthermia during pregnancy?
   a) Cleft palate b) Limb deformities
   c) Neural tube defects d) Polydactyly

40. Which infectious agent is most commonly associated with fetal mummification in cattle?
   a) Toxoplasma gondii b) Brucella abortus
   c) Bovine viral diarrhea virus d) E. coli

41. Congenital heart defects are often associated with exposure to which type of teratogen?
   a) Radiation b) Viral infections
   c) Lead d) Iron deficiency

42. Which condition occurs when the neural tube fails to close at the cranial end?
   a) Spina bifida b) Microcephaly
   c) Anencephaly d) Hydrocephalus

43. Teratology includes the study of which of the following?
   a) Fetal growth rates b) Congenital malformations
   c) Normal embryonic development d) Behavior of neonates

44. Toxoplasmosis in pregnant animals is associated with which type of teratogenic effect?
   a) Skeletal malformations
   b) Fetal abortion or neurological defects
   c) Cardiovascular defects
   d) Cleft palate

45. Micromelia refers to:
   a) Small limbs b) Missing limbs
   c) Extra limbs d) Large limbs

46. Which environmental factor is associated with increased incidence of skeletal malformations in reptiles?
   a) Hyperthermia b) Humidity
   c) Ultraviolet light d) Temperature fluctuation

47. A major cause of cerebellar hypoplasia in calves is infection with which virus?
   a) Feline panleukopenia virus b) Bovine viral diarrhea virus
   c) Bluetongue virus d) Rabies virus

48. Which of the following congenital conditions can be caused by genetic factors as well as teratogens?
 a) Micromelia b) Anencephaly
 c) Cleft palate d) Polydactyly
49. What is the primary effect of prenatal nicotine exposure in animals?
 a) Cardiovascular defects b) Neural tube defects
 c) Eye malformations d) Limb malformations
50. Which of the following can lead to mummification of fetuses in animals?
 a) Genetic mutations b) Bacterial infections
 c) Protozoal infections d) Viral infections
51. What is polydactyly?
 a) Missing limbs b) Extra digits
 c) Fused limbs d) Large limbs
52. Which of the following is a known teratogen that can cause blindness in calves?
 a) Lead b) Vitamin A deficiency
 c) Toxoplasma gondii d) Rubella virus
53. What is the most common teratogenic effect of hyperthermia during early embryonic development?
 a) Cleft palate b) Limb deformities
 c) Neural tube defects d) Skeletal malformations
54. Which chemical exposure during pregnancy can lead to the development of cleft palate in animals?
 a) Nicotine b) Aspirin
 c) Corticosteroids d) Lead
55. Syndactyly refers to which type of congenital abnormality?
 a) Fused digits b) Extra digits
 c) Short limbs d) Absent limbs
56. Folic acid supplementation in pregnant animals helps prevent:
 a) Limb malformations b) Neural tube defects
 c) Cleft palate d) Polydactyly
57. Omphalocele is a congenital defect characterized by:
 a) Brain malformations b) Abnormal eye development
 c) Herniation of abdominal organs d) Missing digit\s
58. Which of the following is a viral teratogen that causes congenital defects in pigs?
 a) Feline parvovirus b) Porcine parvovirus
 c) Canine parvovirus d) Rabies virus
59. Which congenital condition is characterized by failure of the roof of the mouth to close completely?
 a) Cleft palate b) Spina bifida
 c) Omphalocele d) Polydactyly

60. Which virus is known to cause hydrocephalus and porencephaly in ruminant fetuses?
    a) Bluetongue virus
    b) Bovine herpesvirus
    c) Schmallenberg virus
    d) Rabies virus

61. Which teratogen is associated with the formation of ocular malformations in calves?
    a) Lead
    b) Rubella virus
    c) Bluetongue virus
    d) Vitamin A deficiency

62. A defect characterized by the incomplete formation of the skull and brain is called:
    a) Spina bifida
    b) Anencephaly
    c) Hydrocephalus
    d) Cleft palate

63. Which substance is known to cause skeletal malformations in developing animals when deficient?
    a) Vitamin D
    b) Vitamin C
    c) Folic acid
    d) Iron

64. Which of the following is a teratogenic plant that affects the central nervous system of developing embryos in livestock?
    a) Lupine
    b) Nightshade
    c) Hemlock
    d) Veratrum californicum

65. Which congenital defect is characterized by failure of the spinal cord to develop properly?
    a) Anencephaly
    b) Polydactyly
    c) Spina bifida
    d) Hydrocephalus

66. Which of the following congenital malformations is most commonly seen with thalidomide exposure in animals?
    a) Cardiac defects
    b) Limb malformations
    c) Eye defects
    d) Neural tube defects

67. Congenital deafness is often associated with which teratogen in animals?
    a) Lead
    b) Rubella virus
    c) Folic acid deficiency
    d) Aminoglycosides

68. Which virus can cause brain malformations, including microencephaly, in animals?
    a) Canine distemper virus
    b) Bluetongue virus
    c) Feline leukemia virus
    d) Zika virus

69. What is the common teratogenic effect of maternal iodine deficiency in animals?
    a) Goiter
    b) Blindness
    c) Microencephaly
    d) Polydactyly

70. Which nutrient deficiency during pregnancy is most likely to result in skeletal deformities in animals?
    a) Calcium
    b) Vitamin D
    c) Folic acid
    d) Iron

71. Which virus is associated with fetal cerebellar hypoplasia in cattle?
   a) Bluetongue virus b) Bovine viral diarrhea virus
   c) Rabies virus d) Canine parvovirus
72. What is the term for a congenital defect that involves multiple body systems?
   a) Malformation syndrome b) Dysplasia
   c) Teratogenic complex d) Syndactyly
73. Which of the following congenital malformations is commonly seen in kittens whose mothers are infected with feline panleukopenia virus during pregnancy?
   a) Cerebellar hypoplasia b) Spina bifida
   c) Cleft palate d) Hydrocephalus
74. Which drug is associated with limb reduction defects in developing embryos?
   a) Penicillin b) Thalidomide
   c) Corticosteroids d) Aspirin
75. Which term refers to the condition where part of the skull and brain are absent?
   a) Hydrocephalus b) Microencephaly
   c) Anencephaly d) Spina bifida
76. Which infectious agent can cause hydrocephalus and microphthalmia in animals?
   a) Bluetongue virus b) Toxoplasma gondii
   c) Brucella abortus d) E. coli
77. Which of the following conditions is caused by failure of the neural tube to close?
   a) Anencephaly b) Omphalocele
   c) Cleft palate d) Hydrocephalus
78. What is the most common teratogenic effect of maternal diabetes in animals?
   a) Polydactyly b) Cardiac defects
   c) Neural tube defects d) Cleft palate
79. Which type of defect occurs when the limbs are underdeveloped or absent?
   a) Syndactyly b) Micromelia
   c) Amelia d) Polydactyly
80. Which virus is a common teratogen causing neural and eye defects in developing pig fetuses?
   a) Porcine parvovirus b) Swine influenza virus
   c) Rabies virus d) Bovine viral diarrhea virus
81. Which plant is associated with congenital defects such as cleft palate and joint malformations in animals?
   a) Veratrum californicum b) Lupine
   c) Hemlock d) Nightshade
82. What is the effect of congenital rubella infection on developing fetuses in animals?
   a) Cardiovascular defects b) Skeletal malformations
   c) Cleft palate d) Blindness

83. Which congenital condition involves incomplete fusion of the upper lip and roof of the mouth?
   a) Cleft palate b) Polydactyly
   c) Hydrocephalus d) Omphalocele
84. Which teratogen can lead to congenital skeletal malformations in animals?
   a) Radiation b) Folic acid deficiency
   c) Hyperthermia d) Nicotine
85. Which virus is known to cause cerebellar hypoplasia and other neurological defects in calves?
   a) Bovine viral diarrhea virus b) Bluetongue virus
   c) Feline panleukopenia virus d) Canine distemper virus
86. Which of the following describes the impact of a teratogen?
   a) Causes genetic mutations
   b) Inhibits immune function
   c) Disrupts normal embryonic development
   d) Increases the size of the fetus
87. Which nutrient deficiency is associated with neural tube defects in developing embryos?
   a) Vitamin C b) Vitamin D
   c) Folic acid d) Iron
88. What is the impact of congenital Toxoplasma gondii infection in livestock?
   a) Cardiac defects b) Neurological abnormalities
   c) Limb deformities d) Polydactyly
89. Which type of defect involves the absence of limbs?
   a) Polydactyly b) Amelia
   c) Syndactyly d) Cleft palate
90. Which virus is most commonly associated with teratogenic effects in cattle?
   a) Bluetongue virus b) Bovine viral diarrhea virus
   c) Rabies virus d) Canine parvovirus
91. Which plant is associated with the formation of neural tube defects in livestock?
   a) Lupine b) Veratrum californicum
   c) Hemlock d) Nightshade
92. Which congenital abnormality results from the incomplete closure of the neural tube in the lumbar region?
   a) Spina bifida b) Anencephaly
   c) Hydrocephalus d) Polydactyly
93. Which congenital defect is characterized by a failure of the heart to develop properly?
   a) Cardiac septal defect b) Microcephaly
   c) Spina bifida d) Cleft palate

94. What is the result of maternal exposure to high doses of corticosteroids during pregnancy?
a) Blindness b) Neural tube defects
c) Cleft palate d) Heart defects

95. Which virus causes fetal infection that results in cerebellar hypoplasia in kittens?
a) Feline panleukopenia virus b) Rabies virus
c) Canine parvovirus d) Feline leukemia virus

96. What is the most common teratogenic effect of maternal alcohol consumption in animals?
a) Neural tube defects b) Limb malformations
c) Heart defects d) Microencephaly

97. Which teratogen can cause blindness in the offspring of affected animals?
a) Lead b) Vitamin A deficiency
c) Corticosteroids d) Folic acid

98. Which congenital condition involves abnormal development of the neural crest cells?
a) Cleft palate b) Spina bifida
c) Neurocristopathy d) Hydrocephalus

99. Which nutrient deficiency can lead to congenital skeletal deformities in animals?
a) Calcium b) Iron
c) Vitamin D d) Folic acid

100. Which virus can cause microphthalmia and hydrocephalus in infected fetuses?
a) Bluetongue virus b) Porcine parvovirus
c) Rabies virus d) Canine parvovirus

Answer Key

1	b	2	c	3	b	4	c	5	b	6	b	7	b
8	c	9	b	10	b	11	b	12	b	13	a	14	a
15	b	16	c	17	c	18	d	19	b	20	b	21	d
22	b	23	b	24	d	25	a	26	b	27	c	28	a
29	b	30	b	31	c	32	a	33	b	34	b	35	a
36	b	37	b	38	a	39	c	40	c	41	b	42	c
43	b	44	b	45	a	46	a	47	b	48	c	49	a
50	d	51	b	52	b	53	c	54	c	55	a	56	b
57	c	58	b	59	a	60	c	61	d	62	b	63	a
64	a	65	c	66	b	67	d	68	d	69	a	70	b
71	b	72	a	73	a	74	b	75	c	76	b	77	a
78	b	79	c	80	a	81	b	82	a	83	a	84	c
85	a	86	c	87	c	88	b	89	b	90	b	91	b
92	a	93	a	94	c	95	a	96	d	97	b	98	c
99	c	100	a										

27

Assisted Reproduction and Technologies

Jasvinder Singh Sasan, Shalini Suri and Kamal Sarma

Division of Veterinary Anatomy, Faculty of Veterinary Sciences and Animal Husbandry Sher-e-Kashmir University of Agricultural Sciences and Technology of Jammu, Jammu and Kashmir

Introduction

Assisted reproductive technology (ART) refers to treatments and procedures in the field of reproductive biology that are utilised to achieve pregnancy by artificial or partially artificial means.

Artificial insemination

Artificial insemination (AI) is the earliest form of assisted reproductive technology. The technology has been of immense relevance in enhancing production and health features through the appropriate use of better male animals, as well as in eliminating certain venereal illnesses.

- Semen collection: The man is typically allowed to mount a phantom during the process. In cattle, an artificial vagina is used)
- Semen evaluation: Evaluating semen is crucial before processing. The most basic semen evaluation involves examining the concentration, progressive motility, and morphological normality of the spermatozoa)
- Semen dilution, packaging and freezing: Following examination, the semen is ready for dilution and packaging. Spermatozoa require storage mediums that are particular to each species. After packaging, the semen dosages must be properly maintained until insemination. Cryopreservation is typically used for cattle.
- Insemination: Insemination should occur during the female's oestrus, when she is receptive to copulation.

Multiple Ovulation and Embryo Transfer (MOET)

The main processes are to stimulate a donor female to create suitable embryos, then remove the embryos from her and transfer them to unmated recipient females at equivalent post-ovulatory reproductive phases, ensuring that the donor's embryos are carried to term in the recipients' uteri. Multiple ovulations are caused by superovulation or superstimulation, a procedure that increases the number of ovulations in a donor beyond what is normal for a given species. Embryos are recovered 6-8 days following the start of oestrus. Most embryos are transferred during the late morula or blastocyst stage.

In Vitro Fertilization

Bovine embryo production involves three steps: in vitro maturation (IVM), oocyte fertilisation (IVF), and embryo culture (IVc). Despite these three independent processes, the word 'IVF' is frequently used generally to refer to the whole process.

Multiple Choice Questions

1. Among following, the oldest assisted reproduction technology is:
   a) Multiple ovulation embryo transfer b) In vitro fertilization
   c) Artificial insemination d) Ovum pick-up
2. 1st member of horse family to be cloned is:
   a) Snuppy b) Idaho Gem
   c) Virgil d) Frosty
3. 1st cloned dog is:
   a) Snuppy b) Idaho Gem
   c) Virgil d) Frosty
4. 1st member of the horse family to be cloned from an adult cell is:
   a) Frosty b) Prometea born
   c) Louise Brown d) Virgil
5. Development of 'ovum pick-up' in cattle in:
   a) 1989 b) 1996
   c) 1985 d) 1969
6. 1st calf born after IVF is:
   a) Snuppy b) Virgil
   c) Louise Brown d) Prima
7. 1st human baby born following IVF is:
   a) Snuppy b) Virgil
   c) Louise Brown d) Prima
8. Who among the following is credited with carrying out the first embryo transfer in 1890 using rabbits:
   a) Walter Heape b) Haeckel
   c) Pander d) Karl Von Baer
9. Multiple ovulation embryo transfer (MOET) consists of following steps. The correct sequence of these steps is:
   i. Synchronisation of the oestrous cycles of the donor and recipient females
   ii. AI of the donor
   iii. Recovery of embryos from the donor
   iv. Induction of superovulation in the donor
   v. Transfer of embryos to recipients or cryopreservation of the embryos for future transfer
   a) i, ii, iii, iv, v b) ii, i, v, iii, iv
   c) v, i, ii, iii, iv d) i, iv, ii, iii, v

10. The first human conceived following IVF, Louise Brown, was born in:
    a) 1978 b) 1989
    c) 1998 d) 1969
11. The first calf produced by IVF was born in:
    a) 1978 b) 2001
    c) 1981 d) 1990
12. The in vitro production of bovine embryos involves:
    a) Oocyte maturation b) Oocyte fertilization
    c) Embryo culture d) All of the above
13. First mammal produced by IVF was:
    a) Calf b) Mouse
    c) Rabbit d) Monkey
14. Most ideal method of oocyte collection from ovaries is:
    a) Slicing of ovaries b) Follicle aspiration
    c) Follicle puncturing d) None of the above
15. Which of the following media is used for maturation of oocytes:
    a) DMEM b) TCM-199
    c) Ham's F-10 d) Both b & c
16. Which of the following is the indicator of oocyte maturation:
    a) Polar bodies in peri-vitelline space b) Cumulus expansion
    c) Germinal vesicle break down d) All of the above
17. Which of the following is not supplemented with in vitro maturation media:
    a) Estradiol b) FSH
    c) LH d) Progestetone
18. In ICSI, the sperm is injected in:
    a) Cytoplasm b) Nucleoplasm
    c) Perivitelline space d) None of the above
19. Which of the following species oocytes and embryos are highly susceptible to cryodamage:
    a) Buffalo b) Sheep
    c) Goat d) Swine
20. In HMC cloning technique which enzyme is commonly used for digesting zona pellucida:
    a) Pepsin b) Hyaluronidase
    c) Pronase d) Trypsin
21. Which of the following is the first transgenic animal:
    a) Goat b) Mice
    c) Rabbit d) Monkey

22. Conducting a research trial on cloned animals is better than non-cloned animals due to:
    a) Absolute phenotypic control
    b) Absolute genotypic control
    c) Both a & b
    d) Easy availability
23. In cloning protocols while performing ennucleation which chemical is used for relaxing cellular cytoskeleton:
    a) Heparin
    b) Pronase
    c) Cytochalasin B
    d) Phytohaemagglutinin
24. Which of the following is embryo sexing method:
    a) HY antigens
    b) PCR
    c) G6PDH activity
    d) All of the above
25. Which of the following cloning technique renders zona pellucida intact:
    a) HMC
    b) SCNT
    c) Both a & b
    d) None of the above
26. Which embryo stage is preferred for embryo transfer in cloning protocols:
    a) Late blastocyst
    b) Early blastocyst
    c) Late morula
    d) Both b & c
27. In cloning, donor somatic cells should be in which stage of cell cycle:
    a) G0
    b) S
    c) G1
    d) G2
28. Large offspring syndrome is associated with:
    a) IVF
    b) Cloning
    c) Both a & b
    d) None of the above
29. Normal ejaculate occurs in fractions in all of the following except:
    a) Stallion
    b) Bull
    c) Boar
    d) Dog
30. During Multiple ovulation and embryo transfer (MOET) in cattle, donor is injected with drug having:
    a) LH like activity
    b) FSH like activity
    c) Both a & b
    d) None of the above
31. Which of the following is not a step in MOET:
    a) Fertilized eggs are transferred to surrogate mother at 8-32 celled stage
    b) Cow yields 6-8 eggs at a time
    c) Cow is fertilized by AI
    d) Cow is administered hormone having LH like activity
32. What technique involves fertilization outside the body of the female:
    a) Intra-uterine fertilization
    b) In-vivo fertilization
    c) In-vitro fertilization
    d) Ex-vivo fertilization

33. What follows IVF:
    a) Coitus
    b) Embryo transfer
    c) Embryo sacrifice
    d) Embryo delivery
34. ET stands for:
    a) Ejaculate Transfer
    b) Embryo Transfer
    c) Embryo Termination
    d) Embryo Teleportation
35. ZIFT is an acronym for:
    a) zygote intra fallopian transfer
    b) zygote inter fallopian transfer
    c) zygote intra fallopian traction
    d) zygote inter fallopian traction
36. GIFT is an acronym for:
    a) gamete intra fallopian transfer
    b) gamete inter fallopian transfer
    c) gamete intra fallopian traction
    d) gamete inter fallopian traction
37. What method can be used for carrying out in vivo fertilization for a sterile but fertile female:
    a) ZIFT
    b) GIFT
    c) IUT
    d) AI
38. ICSI stands for:
    a) intra cytoplasmic sperm injection
    b) inter cytoplasmic sperm injection
    c) intra cytoplasmic semen injection
    d) inter cytoplasmic semen injection
39. What technique is used to inject the sperm directly into the ovum in a laboratory setting:
    a) ZIFT
    b) GIFT
    c) IUT
    d) ICSI
40. International Embryo Transfer Society was founded in:
    a) 1974
    b) 1984
    c) 1990
    d) 1965
41. IETS stands for:
    a) Indian Embryo Transfer Society
    b) International Embryo Transfer Society
    c) Italian Embryo Transfer Society
    d) None of the above
42. The first ET piglets were produced in 1950 in:
    a) Japan
    b) USA
    c) Ukraine
    d) UK
43. Injection of Prostaglandin in synchronized recipient to that of donor is:
    a) 1 day later than donor
    b) 1day earlier than donor
    c) Same day
    d) Three days early
44. Superovulatory hormones are injected during:
    a) Early follicular phase
    b) Late Follicular phase
    c) Mid luteal phase
    d) Late luteal phase

45. Calves produced from the cloning process is having:
   a) Smaller than normal calves
   b) 20 % heavier than normal calves
   c) 20 % lighter than normal calves
   d) Both are equal
46. Average recovery of transferable embryos in cattle in each flush is:
   a) 1-2 embryo
   b) 0.5 -1 embryo
   c) 10 – 12 embryo
   d) 3- 7 embryo
47. Average recovery of transferable embryos in buffalo in each flush is:
   a) 1-2 embryo
   b) 0.5 -1 embryo
   c) 10 – 12 embryo
   d) 3- 7 embryo
48. Average sperm concentration in Dog semen is:
   a) 800-1400 million/ml
   b) 600-1200 million/ml
   c) 200-400 million/ml
   d) 2000-4000 million/ml
49. Average sperm concentration in Ram semen is:
   a) 800-1400 million/ml
   b) 600-1200 million/ml
   c) 2000-4000 million/ml
   d) 200-400 million/ml
50. The ideal concentration of glycerol in diluents for the preservation of buffalo bull semen:
   a) 2 %
   b) 6%
   c) 12 %
   d) 18 %
   e) None of these

Answer Key

1	c	2	b	3	a	4	b	5	a	6	b	7	c
8	a	9	d	10	a	11	c	12	d	13	c	14	b
15	d	16	b	17	d	18	a	19	d	20	c	21	b
22	c	23	c	24	d	25	c	26	d	27	a	28	b
29	b	30	b	31	d	32	c	33	b	34	b	35	a
36	a	37	b	38	a	39	d	40	a	41	b	42	c
43	b	44	b	45	c	46	b	47	d	48	c	49	c
50	a												